Social Groupwork
&
Alcoholism

Other titles in the *Social Work with Groups* series:

- *Groupwork with the Frail Elderly*, edited by Shura Saul
- *The Use of Group Services in Permanency Planning for Children*, edited by Beulah Rothman and Catherine P. Papell

Social Groupwork
&
Alcoholism

Marjorie Altman & Ruth Crocker

Guest Editors

Social Work with Groups
Volume 5, Number 1

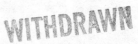

The Haworth Press
New York • London

The Haworth Press, Inc., 12 West 32 Street, New York, NY 10001
EUROSPAN/Haworth, 3 Henrietta Street, London WC2E 8LU England

Library of Congress Cataloging in Publication Data
Main entry under title:

Social groupwork & alcoholism.

(Social work with groups ; v. 5, no. 1)
Bibliography: p.
1. Social work with alcoholics — Addresses, essays, lectures. 2. Social group work — Addresses, essays, lectures. 3. Alcoholism — Treatment — Addresses, essays, lectures. 4. Alcoholics — Family relationships — Addresses, essays, lectures. I. Altman, Marjorie. II. Crocker, Ruth. III. Series: Social work with groups (Haworth Press); v. 5, no. 1.
HV5275.S65   362.2'9254   82-2998
ISBN 0-917724-94-1   AACR2

Social Groupwork & Alcoholism

Social Work with Groups
Volume 5, Number 1

EDITORIAL

The flow of papers across the Editor's Desk of any professional journal provides an indication of the cutting edge of professional practice, or points up the gaps in knowledge necessary to generate or sustain new directions for practice. The Special Issue is a response to such identifiable trends in professional interest and in the need for professional knowledge building.

We are pleased that two colleagues, both distinguished practitioners in the field of alcoholism, Marjorie Altman and Ruth Crocker agreed to organize this special issue of *Social Work with Groups*. Their understanding of the multiple and intergenerational reverberations of the disease of alcoholism at all levels of society is reflected in their selection of papers for this issue on the use of groups in treatment and preventive services.

The emphasis on health of our guest editors and their panel of advisors in considering the illness of alcoholism suggests their firm connection with the traditions of Social Work and specifically social group work.

This issue is one of several to appear in the coming year that we hope will extend the contribution of the journal to our readers, old and new.

CP
BR

Guest Editors and Advisory Panel for Volume 5, Number 1

GUEST EDITORS

MARJORIE ALTMAN, CSW, *Social Worker, Family Treatment, Out-Patient Department, Smithers Alcohol Treatment and Training Center, St. Luke's Roosevelt Hospital, New York, NY*
RUTH CROCKER, CSW, *Deputy Director, Long Island Council on Alcoholism, Mineola, NY*

ADVISORY PANEL

GERALD HOROWITZ, CSW, *Supervisor, Out-Patient Department, Smithers Alcohol Treatment Center, St. Luke's Roosevelt Hospital, New York, NY*
HON. VINCENT McCONNELL, JS, LLM, *Judge of the Family Court, City of New York*

ELLEN MOREHOUSE, CSW, *Director, School-Based Prevention Program, Department of Community Mental Health, White Plains, NY*
ROBERT O'CONNOR, MD, *Medical Director, Chit Chat Farms, Wernersville, PA*
NATALIE SALTZMAN, MS, CSW, *Consultant on Aging, Associates for Living and Learning, Roslyn, NY*

GUEST EDITORIAL

Alcoholics have, for years, thwarted the attempts of people to help them. They have confounded professionals with their resistance, their lack of insight, their failure to respond to treatment. In the eyes of social workers and most other helping people, they have been frustrating patients who failed appointments, did not pay their bills, and refused to get well.

With the advent of Alcoholics Anonymous in 1935, some began to achieve sobriety. As membership in this mysterious society grew, more alcoholics recovered. They stopped drinking and either resumed or started satisfying ways of living. However, many continued to appear in physical and mental health offices, and continued to drive therapists crazy. Skilled professionals who treated alcoholics on a one-to-one basis wondered why they failed despite their best efforts, and what A. A. had that they did not.

The most significant answer lies in the use of group. Actively drinking alcoholics are isolated people with virtually no positive self-image. They are loners who, when they can begin to interact with other recovering alcoholics, discover a common bond. As interpersonal communication replaces isolation, hope, acceptance and a sense of belonging dispel loneliness.

Over the last ten years, groups for alcoholics and their families have burgeoned in professional settings, with an impressive increase in successful treatment. A. A. and professional treatment in combination are entirely compatible. As discrete treatment modalities, they complement each other. Many alcoholics require skilled services in addition to A. A. to work through their problems in early sobriety, and often find they do best with this dual treatment approach.

When we were invited to be guest editors for this special issue of *Social Work with Groups*, we accepted out of our conviction that the problems of alcoholism are general to the population and specific to the field of social work. We welcomed the opportunity to add our expertise to the body of knowledge on social group work. All social workers are familiar with alcoholism in its extreme manifestations. They *see* the adverse effects on individuals, nuclear and extended families, and all others in the alcoholic's system. Unfortunately, many do not see recovery. We feel it is vital for all workers in the helping professions to be sensitive to the possibility of recovery and to the treatment modalities that best foster it.

Health is the focus of this issue. The papers that follow describe a variety of groups that advance, by interpersonal means, the goals of sobriety for alcoholics and a corresponding return to health for family members and all significant others. To cite only a few, Cohen and Spinner discuss a comprehensive outpatient program, Balis and Zirpoli a short-term, hospital-based family program, Brown and Sunshine a group for latency-age children of alcoholic parents, and Rothfeld an innovative treatment for deaf alcoholics. There are many segments of the drinking population, and many excellent treatment facilities, that could not be covered in these pages, but we hope the readers will finish reading this issue with a new awareness of the value of group work in the treatment of alcoholism.

Marjorie Altman
Ruth Crocker

A GROUP CURRICULUM FOR OUTPATIENT ALCOHOLISM TREATMENT

Mark Cohen
Allyne Spinner

ABSTRACT. Although groups are the treatment of choice in many alcoholism programs, they often fail to take into full account the changing needs of the alcoholic during the early stages of recovery. This paper describes a five-phase group curriculum for outpatient alcoholism treatment. The curriculum is unique in that it addresses the changing needs of the alcoholic from active drinking through one year of sobriety by viewing the recovery process as a continuum. This enables clients to build upon strengths acquired during the preceding phase(s). All of the curriculum's phases are consistent with the philosophy of Alcoholics Anonymous, and eventual commitment of the clients to A.A. is one of the program's fundamental objectives. Empirical data on the effectiveness of the curriculum are not yet available; however, it appears thus far to be an extremely helpful tool in outpatient treatment and in maximizing the chances for the alcoholic to maintain long-term sobriety.

The use of homogeneous groups as a therapeutic modality in health care has been common. In many alcoholism treatment settings, groups have evolved into the "treatment of choice," due to the effectiveness of results. The specific dynamics of alcoholism necessitate a variety of groups corresponding to particular stages in the recovery process, each group possessing its own unique purpose, structure, function, and style of leadership.

The absence from the literature of a comprehensive group curriculum dealing with the period from the initiation of treatment through one year of sobriety is clearly apparent. This paper reports on the development and use of a group curriculum for outpatient alcoholism programs, and delineates how each group meets the needs of the alcoholic at varying stages of treat-

Mark Cohen, DSW, MPH, is the Director of Alcoholism Services, and Allyne Spinner, MSW, is Group Supervisor at St. John's Episcopal Hospital Out-Patient Alcoholism Program, Far Rockaway, NY.

The authors wish to thank the staff of the St. John's Out-Patient Alcoholism Program as well as Louis Wheeler and Carol Joyce, whose ideas and creativity contributed to the development of the group curriculum.

ment. Finally, the relationship of the group curriculum to other alcoholism treatment methodologies will be explored.

Background

The health field has used homogeneous groups to enable clients to share common concerns and gain therapeutic benefits through the concept of universality (Pratt, 1907). Frey (1966) contended that homogeneous groups "help members assume responsibility for themselves and handle such emotional responses to illness as depression, guilt, aggression and dependency." Such groups also contribute to the development of positive morale and provide opportunity "for people to discover they are not so odd or different as they think or so alone with their heartaches" (Yeakel, 1966). Homogeneous groups have been commonly used to treat alcoholism because of the widespread success of the group approach of Alcoholics Anonymous (A.A.), the meager achievements of the orthodox psychoanalytic approach in alcoholism, and better understanding of the psychodynamics of the disease (Fox, 1962). Also negative transference toward the leader is diminished in groups because of their diverse nature and the dilution of the therapist's authority by the presence of group members (Hartocollis and Shaefor 1968).

Although there is controversy as to whether there is an alcoholic personality, most alcoholics seem to possess certain characteristics, including low frustration tolerance, inability to endure anxiety, feelings of isolation, devaluated self-esteem, extreme narcissism, poor object relations, obsessive-compulsive traits, punitive superegos, depression, strong dependency needs, problems dealing with anger, and perceptual difficulties including memory and cognition problems. Major defense mechanisms seem to be denial, projection, and rationalization (Fox, 1962). Some authors feel that these psychodynamics can be best addressed therapeutically in a group setting, in which alcoholics can identify common problems that have resulted from excessive drinking (Esser, 1961). Fried (1971) stated that therapeutic benefits of using what she called "supportive homogeneous inspirational groups" in the treatment of alcoholism include peer identification, mutual support, and the idealization of those who maintain sobriety. Lindt (1959) suggested that groups substitute the elation of the group for the euphoric state of drunkenness. Hartocollis and Shaefor (1968) suggested that, because of narcissistic defenses, the alcoholic tends to find it easier to understand the personal problems of other group members than to understand his or her own problems. Later, the alcoholic can comfortably understand him- or herself and can tolerate confrontation from alcoholic peers through partial identification.

The Problem

Group treatment must take the above characteristics into account by keeping anxiety low and by providing structure and repetition, especially in the early phases of treatment. Too much anxiety can lead to drinking, while an absence of structure can perpetuate an irresponsible "alcoholic lifestyle."

The dependency needs of the alcoholic are also met in the beginning of treatment by replacing dependency on alcohol with dependency on group members. Relationships with others help the alcoholic cope with feelings of loneliness, isolation, and devaluated self-esteem. The narcissism and grandiosity of the alcoholic must be redirected (Zimberg, 1978) toward helping others in group. The defense mechanisms of projection, rationalization, and denial should be redirected and built upon but not challenged, especially in the early phases of treatment (Wallace, 1978).

Once an alcoholic obtains sobriety, he or she will start to experience feelings such as anger and depression. Through group process the client will learn how to experience and cope with these feelings without drinking. The later stages of treatment must gradually begin to address the problems of low frustration tolerance, need for immediate gratification, punitive superego, and obsessive-compulsive traits, which if left alone continually threaten sobriety. These personality (characterological) changes are necessary for recovery and are dealt with only after six months to a year of sobriety.

Specific different group techniques for treating alcoholism, such as the Decision Group (Levinson, 1979) and the Psychodrama Group (Weiner, 1965), have been developed. However, a review of the literature shows that an outpatient group curriculum that meets the needs of alcoholics through one year of uninterrupted sobriety has not been developed.

Following is a report on a five-phase curriculum for alcoholic outpatients that has recently been developed and used at a hospital-based program of recovery. It should be noted that while the main treatment modality is groups, other services such as individual counseling, family and marital counseling, vocational counseling, and medical and psychiatric evaluations, are integral program components. Participation in A.A. is strongly encouraged.

The Curriculum

One reason for the use of a phase system is that it sequentially reinforces sobreity. Clients must meet sobriety and other requirements before moving on to the next phase of treatment. A second reason is that the alcoholic's needs change with the length of sobriety.

The groups, attended in consecutive order, are designed to meet the clients' changing needs. Clients move from acquiring information and working on denial and avoidance of problems to accepting their disease. In Phase 5, they work on other problems and feelings that threaten sobriety. They move from getting sober, in early phases, to living sober, in later phases. Groups in the early phases have little feeling content and a lot of structure and repetition. In later phases, there is less structure and more focus on feelings. The early groups also take into account patients' perceptual difficulties and the need for visual aids, repetition, and clarity. The leadership styles change from active involvement in the early phases to less active involvement later on, as patients take on more responsibility. Each phase has a specific purpose, which is shared with the members at the beginning of each group. This is consistent with the social group work "contract," in which group members mutually invest themselves in the common purpose of the group (Tropp, 1969).

Phase 1: Orientation

The orientation group prepares clients for the patient role (Frey, 1966) and introduces new clients to the program and its policies. This group gives clients a beginning group experience in which they can share their reasons for entering treatment. It also introduces them to some facts about alcoholism. The group meets for two one-hour sessions in one week. The sessions are very structured, and the leader is extremely active. Session 1 covers program policies and includes a description of the entire program. Clients share concerns about being in treatment, discuss factors that influenced their seeking treatment, and can express feelings about the program's policies and services. Repetition is common, since some clients have damaged recall due to prolonged alcohol abuse. In Session 2, a film about alcoholism is shown as a catalyst for discussion and to prepare clients for the next phase. Clients can ask questions and share their experience in the program to date, especially if they have attended a selective group or an A.A. meeting. They are encouraged to give feedback about the orientation process. Once a client completes orientation, he or she moves on to Phase 2.

Phase 2: Elementary Alcohol Education

The purpose of Phase 2 is to give clients clear and accurate information about alcohol and alcoholism. According to Fox (1962), in "early treatment the therapy should be didactic and informative. Patients must be taught all we know about the condition, its definition, case, incidence, treatment and prevention. The didactic part can be aided by books and films.'' Alcohol education serves as motivation for actively drinking clients to get sober and for those who are already sober to remain so. This group meets for five one-hour sessions once a week. Each session covers a different topic:

> Session 1: What is alcohol?
> Session 2: What is an alcoholic?
> Session 3: What is alcoholism?
> Session 4: Film (*Chalk Talk*) and discussion.
> Session 5: Treatment modalities and recovery: Film (*The Other Guy*) and discussion.

This is an open group without fixed membership or size. The group is extremely structured, and uses a lecture-discussion format. Leaders are active and encourage interaction among members. Visual aids (films, handouts, and blackboard) are used in recognition of the perceptual difficulties of alcoholics in the early stages of treatment. Clients must complete all five sessions before moving on to the next phase.

Phase 3: Identification*

This phase is designed to address the needs of the active drinker and the newly sober alcoholic. It gives clients a chance to apply the information gained in alcohol education. Clients here identify whether or not they are alcoholic and begin to break down denial and rationalization. They are helped to achieve one month of uninterrupted sobriety. This is the first phase in which group process is the major focus; however, the leader is active and the group remains structured. A list of 50 questions is used by the group to help clients explore and personalize behavior characteristics of alcoholism as it assists them in confronting one another. Some of these questions are:

1. Do you think you are an alcoholic and why?
2. Did you ever have a blackout?
3. Do you make promises to yourself about cutting down on drinking which you do not keep?
4. Do you find it easier to confront someone who has done something to bother you, when you have been drinking?
5. Has drinking affected your reputation?

---

*The concept of an identification group was developed at the Bedford-Stuyvesant Alcoholism Treatment Center, Brooklyn, NY.

Through these questions and the responses to them, clients discuss their feelings about drinking and being alcoholic. The questions to be discussed at each session are selected by the leader.

Each session is one hour long, and the group meets weekly. Size is limited to 15. A client may begin at any time and must attend 12 sessions. Having achieved one month of sobriety, and perceived oneself as alcoholic, the client moves on to the next phase. Some people stay in this phase for more than 12 weeks because they are having difficulty attaining one month of sobriety. If they are unable to proceed further they are often referred to inpatient rehabilitation for more intensive treatment.

In this phase the group leader is a recovering alcoholic and serves as a role model. The leader shares his or her experiences in drinking and in achieving and maintaining sobriety. It is the leader's responsibility to keep the group focused on the questions while facilitating client interaction, confrontation, and the sharing of experiences.

Phase 4: Theme Group—Living Sober

The theme group helps clients maintain sobriety by working through common problems of the early stages of recovery, which are reflected in the "themes" for each meeting. A second purpose is helping clients examine and explore feelings about sobriety in a nonthreatening way, which prepares them for entering the last phase of the program. The theme group meets once a week for ten weeks, and each session lasts 1½ hours. The group is closed, which enables clients to share their feelings in an intimate setting for the first time in the program. The members make a verbal contract to come to all ten sessions. Those who do not attend a minimum of eight of the ten must repeat Phase 4. (The reinforcement of responsibility is one ingredient in the maintenance of sobriety.)

The group is limited to ten to twelve members. The topics for the meeting are arranged sequentially, but group leaders have the option of altering the order. The themes, in the order in which they are usually discussed, are (1) the rewards and expectations of sobriety, (2) the stigma of being an alcoholic, (3) depression, (4) holidays, (5) anger, (6) dealing with criticism, (7) loneliness and socializing, (8) fear, (9) love, and (10) endings. Group members share feelings about themselves in relation to the topic, and the leader keeps the group focused on the topic for the session.

A member who returns to drinking while in this phase is expected to discuss this with the group. The client then returns to Phase 3 until one month of sobriety has again been achieved. This policy is explained in the first group session, but clients' feelings about it are often not expressed until a member "has a slip." The leader then re-emphasizes that the theme group is designed for sober people and that individuals who are drinking need to focus on getting sober; consequently, they are best served by the Phase 3 group.

Phase 5: Group Therapy

This phase enables recovering alcoholics to share their everyday concerns and help one another maintain sobriety. In addition, the group helps clients work through personality difficulties, personal problems, and unresolved issues that may or may not be directly related to their alcoholism. As such, the purpose, structure, and function of this phase resembles those of many traditional group therapies.

The group is ongoing and has no time limit. It has a maximum of ten members. New members are assigned to an existing therapy group; however, if there are more members ready for group therapy than there are spaces in existing groups, a new group is formed.

There is no specified agenda. Members make a contract to put their thoughts and feelings into words, and agree to not eat or smoke during sessions to further facilitate talking (Ormont, 1962). The focus is usually on the "here and now," although issues of conflict from the past can also be discussed. Feelings are expected to be dealt with and personalized in more depth than in previous groups. The worker facilitates the group process and helps members get in touch with and work through their real feelings while they acquire additional coping skills. This group deals with the realities of living sober; drinking issues as such are secondary. However, the group is not analytic, and thus unconscious processes are not the focal point. The same rule that applied to Phase 4 regarding drinking is applicable here, except that three months of sobriety and completion of the theme group are needed to rejoin Phase 5. Clients complete Phase 5 when the group worker, the client's counselor and supervisor, and the client feel that the treatment goals have been realized, and when a minimum of one year of uninterrupted sobriety has been attained.

Use of the Group Curriculum

This group curriculum has been in use for two years. During this time the phases have undergone some modification and refinement based on the experience of those working with the curriculum on a regular basis. Consequently, an empirical analysis to substantiate successful treatment using this particular curriculum is so far unavailable. However, the experience to date strongly suggests that the curriculum is therapeutically sound and clinically advantageous—a substantial number of alcoholics have completed the third phase of the program with a minimum of one year of uninterrupted sobriety.

A major asset of the curriculum is its flexibility, which allows the group leaders to make adjustments when circumstances warrant. The curriculum can be modified if it is determined that a specific subgroup has unique needs. For example, if an outpatient clinic has a large number of patients with organic brain syndrome or another type of cognitive disorder, Phase 2 (alcohol education) can be modified so that less information is provided and more repetition is used, thereby making it easier to comprehend. Similarly, the number of sessions in this phase can be expanded. Irrespective of the change(s), the basic principles of the curriculum remain constant and the progression of the treatment is unaltered.

Advantages of the Group Curriculum

The essential strength of the group curriculum is its relevance to the changing needs of the alcoholic at different points in the recovery process. It seems to be a particularly appropriate model for the rebuilding of a sober, more self-sustaining, responsible individual. Although this group curriculum is developmentally in its formative stages, the same can be said for all alcoholism treatment models, in that treatment of this disease is in its infancy. The group curriculum model utilizes some of the principles and treatment philosophies of A.A. and encourages outpatients to become actively involved in A.A. Examples of the A.A. principles utilized are (1) the view of alcoholism as a disease, (2) the commitment to total abstinence, (3) sharing of common problems, and (4) recognizing and taking responsibility for one's character defects. The group acts as an adjunct but does not replace A.A. Clients are not considered ready for termination from the outpatient alcoholism program until they have been soundly integrated into A.A.

REFERENCES

Esser, P.M. Group psychotherapy with alcoholics. *Quarterly Journal of Studies on Alcohol,* 1961, *22,* 4.

Fox, R. Group psychotherapy with alcoholics. *International Journal of Group Psychotherapy,* 1962, *12,* 1.

Frey, L. (Ed.), *Use of groups in the health field.* New York, National Association of Social Workers, 1966.

Fried, E. Basic concepts in group psychotherapy. In Kaplan, H.I., & Sadock, B.J. (Eds.), *Comprehensive group psychotherapy.* Baltimore, Williams and Wilkins, 1971.

Hartocollis, P., & Shaefor, D. Group psychotherapy with alcoholics: A critical review. *Psychiatry Digest,* 1968, *29,* 6.

Levinson, V. The decision group. *Health and Social Work*, 1979, *4*, 4.

Lindt, H. The rescue fantasy in group treatment of alcoholics. *International Journal of Group Psychotherapy*, 1959, *9*, 1.

Ormont, L. Establishing the analytic contract in a newly formed therapeutic group. *British Journal of Medical Psychology*, 1962, *35*, 4.

Pratt, J.H. The class method of treating consumption in the homes of the poor. *Journal of American Medical Association*, 1907, *49*, 1.

Tropp, E. A humanistic view of social group work. In *A humanistic foundation for group work practice*. New York, Simon and Schuster, 1969.

Wallace, J. The preferred defense structure of the alcoholic. In Zimberg, S., Wallace, J., & Blume, S. (Eds.), *Practical approaches to alcoholism psychotherapy*. New York, Plenum Press, 1978.

Weiner, H. Treating the alcoholic with psychodrama. *Group Psychotherapy*, 1965, *18*, 1-2.

Yeakel, M. Theoretical considerations. In Frey, L. (Ed.), *Use of groups in the health field*, New York, National Association of Social Workers, 1966.

Zimberg, S. Principles of alcoholism psychotherapy, and Treatment of socioeconomically deprived alcoholics. In Zimberg, S., Wallace, J. & Blume, S. (Eds.), *Practical approaches to alcoholism psychotherapy*. New York: Plenum Press, 1978.

S.O.B.E.R.:
A STRESS MANAGEMENT PROGRAM
FOR RECOVERING ALCOHOLICS

Alan Brody

ABSTRACT. This paper will describe the S.O.B.E.R. program as a way to bridge the gap between our knowledge about stress control and the needs of the recovering alcoholic. It does this by providing an approach to stress management that can be integrated into the alcoholism recovery program of Alcoholics Anonymous. The approach is a cognitive-behavioral one, since treatment is founded on the principle that a person's emotional and behavioral reactions are determined by a person's cognitive behavior.

This paper describes a stress management program for recovering alcoholics. The treatment modality used is based on the principles and techniques of cognitive-behavior therapy (Beck, 1976; Ellis, 1962; Mahoney, 1974; Meichenbaum, 1977). Although a few practitioners have relied on cognitive-behavioral procedures in treating alcoholics (Ellis, 1973; Criddle, 1977; Grau, 1977; Higbee, 1977; Hindman, 1976; Jackson & Oei, 1978; McCourt & Glantz, 1980; Sanchez-Craig, 1975; Snyder, 1975), their methods have not been integrated into a program specifically designed for teaching stress-management skills to recovering alcoholics. This paper concerns itself with describing such a program.

The S.O.B.E.R. program is a treatment package that the author originated and implemented in group settings at the Smithers Center for Alcoholism Treatment, St. Luke's Roosevelt Hospital. "S.O.B.E.R." is an acronym in which each letter signifies a step in managing stress reactions such as anxiety, tension, panic, and feeling worried, pressured, and overwhelmed. The aim of the program is to foster coping with stress without resorting to mood-altering drugs.

Incorporated into the teaching of S.O.B.E.R. are the examination of the following: (1) various stress management procedures; (2) attitudes and

---

Alan Brody, CSW, PhD, is a social worker at Smithers Alcoholism Treatment and Training Center, St. Luke's Roosevelt Hospital Center, New York, NY.

behaviors responsible for either engendering or reducing stress; (3) interpretations, relevant to managing stress, of Alcoholics Anonymous (A.A.)
slogans such as "Easy does it," "First things first," "Don't project," "Turn
it over," "Just for today," and the famous Serenity Prayer; (4) how to handle
barriers that may arise in being able to effectively apply the knowledge and
skills taught; and (5) the integration of the above knowledge and skills into
a systematized set of procedures serving as a personalized guide for managing
stress.

Some of the principles and techniques of S.O.B.E.R. can be found in
other stress management treatment approaches and programs (Ellis & Harper,
1977; Meichenbaum & Turk, 1976; Novaco, 1978; Suinn & Richardson,
1971). However, they have not concentrated on designing their programs
with the needs of the recovering alcoholic in mind. One program that does
take the recovering alcoholic's needs seriously is A.A., but it is designed
to help people stay sober rather than to provide an organized stress management program.

The S.O.B.E.R. program is a way to bridge the gap between our
knowledge about stress control and the needs of the recovering alcoholic.
It does this by providing an approach to stress management that can be integrated into the alcoholism recovery program of A.A. The approach is a
cognitive-behavioral one, since treatment is founded on the principle that
a person's emotional and behavioral reactions are determined by a person's
cognitive behavior. Modification of the latter results in modification of the
former (Ellis, 1962; Beck, 1976). The uniqueness and value of S.O.B.E.R.
are due to the originality and/or use of certain stress management principles
and procedures, the way they are integrated with the A.A. program, and
the creation of a new group of coping skills that can be implemented in
alcoholism programs.

The usefulness of S.O.B.E.R. to recovering alcoholics is enhanced when
it is taught within a group context, which allows the individual to hear about
the success that others have had using stress management skills. This is
a valuable experience for someone who finds it very difficult to believe that
there can be alternatives to alcohol or other mood-altering drugs in dealing
with stress. By example and direct confrontation, group members challenge
the belief that alcohol (or some other mood-altering drug) is necessary for
stress reduction and relaxation. In S.O.B.E.R., alibis for using chemicals
that appeal to the person's "intolerable" level of stress (e.g., "I just couldn't
stand the anxiety") are powerfully confronted by peers who know how to
challenge those excuses.

In summary, S.O.B.E.R. provides access to some powerful means of breaking through certain resistances to change. Sobriety is strengthened via (1) decreasing the ability of stress to trigger a relapse; (2) increasing the quality of that sobriety, and (3) fostering A.A. involvement. In addition, a person who has learned to trust his or her ability to handle stress will experience greater self-esteem, which in turn, increases motivation to remain sober. Since different groups may have different needs and abilities, the principles and methods of S.O.B.E.R. will be described without suggesting a timetable to be followed for presenting the material. It will be left to the discretion of the clinician to structure the term of the group.

Introductory Phase

The first session typically opens with a statement of the purpose, duration, and nature of the group. Members are encouraged to voice their expectations. It is important that the members realize they will be learning skills that are acquired over time and that there may be times when they will have difficulty applying the tools to reduce stress. It should also be added that, with commitment and sustained practice, group members will become increasingly proficient at handling stress. Incorporated into this introductory phase of the program is a discussion about the signs of stress (anxiety, tension, "butterflies" in the stomach, headaches, muscle pains, rapid heart beat, dry mouth, sweaty palms, difficulty concentrating, etc.). Members are encouraged to verbalize their typical stress reactions.

All group members will probably be able to identify with the description of a person who is experiencing an anxiety reaction, whether due to fear of talking at A.A. meetings, going for a job interview, or being in any other particularly uncomfortable situation. The person's mind races with alarming thoughts of how things did not, or will not, work out. The person describes the experience in terms such as "awful," "terrible," "horrible," "unbearable," etc. There may be physical manifestations of anxiety, such as sweating, palpitations, difficulty breathing, and the person worries about their getting worse. The individual may pace, speak and respond, quickly, as if he or she is burning excess nervous energy. The person's perception of his or her own anxiety reaction produces alarming cognitions about that reaction ("How much more can I take?") such that more anxiety is generated. By this point, the individual is caught up in an escalating cycle of stress. Examples like the one above will help the members of S.O.B.E.R. become aware that their thoughts and behaviors have an important role in provoking physical stress responses.

The "S" Step

The group is now ready to learn how to intervene in the stress cycle. At the very first signs of stress, before it intensifies and becomes more difficult to handle, members are taught to follow the the first step of S.O.B.E.R. The "S" stands for the self-command, "Stop and slow down," by which method the alarming, agitated flow of thoughts, images, and behaviors is stopped or interrupted. To accomplish this, members are first taught the techniques of thought stopping (Wolpe, 1958). In addition, they are told to pace themselves, that is, to perform cognitive and/or physical activity at a slower or slow pace. The combination of thought stopping and pacing provides a means of behaviorally instituting the slogan, "Easy does it." Thought stopping is usually performed via a covert self-command ("Stop!") or a mental image (a stop sign) that is antagonistic to the flow of stress-engendering behavior. This self-command is covertly repeated until the negative flow of behavior is significantly interfered with. Participants are taught to pace themselves immediately thereafter, so that their behavior does not get out of control or agitated to the point of triggering a full stress reaction.

A.A. members are familiar with the acronym H.A.L.T., which is a reminder not to get too Hungry, Angry, Lonely, or Tired. It is sometimes effective to encourage patients to incorporate this maxim into the covert self-command repertoire acquired during the phase of the program. Members rehearse the procedure after the therapist models it, and are asked to practice it between group sessions. All of the coping skills presented in S.O.B.E.R. are modeled, rehearsed, and practiced.

At the next group session, members share their experiences using the "S" step. Any difficulties encountered in implementing the program are dealt with by the participants. The leader may orchestrate the dialogue with suggestions about other specific techniques, such as mental imagery: patients can imagine a red stop sign or a drill sergeant barking out the "Stop!" Members should be encouraged to develop their ability to slow down their behavior and to continue repeating the coping instructions to themselves. These reminders will be an important part of their learning new coping skills.

The "O" Step

One very useful technique for handling stress is the tension-relaxation exercise (T.R.E.) or progressive relaxation (Jacobson, 1929). In T.R.E. the individual tenses, in sequence, the various muscle groups of the body, and then, after several seconds relaxes them. Calming sensations are experienced as the tensed muscle groups are relaxed.

The "O" in S.O.B.E.R. indicates the taking in of oxygen (air) by deep breathing. This enhances the sensation of relaxation. The patient is enjoined to take a deep breath, hold it, and then slowly exhale. Upon exhalation, a relaxing, calming sensation is felt. To avoid lightheadedness, this procedure is repeated no more than a few times in succession. The deep breathing may be done with or without T.R.E., depending on circumstances. Since the clinician can readily obtain step-by-step instructions on T.R.E. (Bernstein & Borkovec, 1976; Goldfried & Davidson, 1976; Jacobson, 1929; Rimm & Masters, 1979), the procedure will not be detailed further here.

The group participants are taught progressive relaxation as a tool to be used before, during, and after actual stressful events. However, since there may not be sufficient time for the individual to go through the entire procedure during a stressful episode, a highly effective modified version is recommended; this involves deep breathing, alone or in conjunction with a few strategic tension-relaxation exercises, such as relaxing the back muscles.

The patients select their own brief T.R.E. and practice using it in the group sessions. Although between-session practice is encouraged, members are told that daily practice is not necessary for obtaining benefits from T.R.E. (In the author's experience, sustained and regular T.R.E. practice is not achieved by most of the group members.) The experience of failure can be avoided by conceptualizing T.R.E. as a useful coping skill experientially learned and used when appropriate in stress-related situations.

By this time, group members have learned that in a stressful situation they can start coping by using the step and adding the deep breathing with or without T.R.E. (It should be emphasized that S.O.B.E.R. organizes principles for coping, but is *not* a set of rules that must be followed in strict sequence for successful stress management.)

Meditation can be a beneficial adjunct to the methods of step "O" with some patients (Benson, 1975; Carrington, 1978).

The "B.E." Step

A person's self-verbalizations and visual imagery can also cause emotional and physiological arousal (Mahoney, 1974; May & Johnson, 1973; Rimm & Litvak, 1969; Russell & Brandsman, 1974; Schachter, 1966; Schwartz, 1971; Velten, 1968). In the "B.E." (Behavioral exchange) step of the S.O.B.E.R. program, the members learn about the role their cognitions have in mediating stress reactions. In addition, the group examines attitudes about managing stress that foster or impede its amelioration.

The participants begin the "B.E." phase by discussing the thoughts and mental images that occur spontaneously in stress situations. They frequently use terms such as "nightmare," "catastrophe," "disaster," "terrible," "awful," "horrible," and the like in describing the trigger event. They conceptualize the experience in the language of, and with a sense of, alarm. As a result, they feel fear about undergoing or facing such a severe experience. This fear then evokes doubts about the adequacy of their resources in coping with the stressor. Such doubts are often expressed in statements such as "I can't stand it" or "This is driving me crazy." In addition, questions are raised about the stressor, oneself, and one's fate (e.g., "How long will it last?" "Why do I have to go through that?" "When will things get better?"). The person's questions typically involve self-pity and a craving for alarm-reducing reassurances. However, the individual answers the questions in terms of distressing predictions and self-hatred (e.g., "This must be my fault," "It'll last forever," "Things will never improve"). Group members can often recall instances in which negative cognitions triggered a stress reaction, which was subsequently "handled" by use of a mood-altering drug. Once patients familiarize themselves with the different kinds of negative cognitive activities that accompany stress, they can begin to understand the role these thoughts have in creating alibis for drinking under stress (e.g., "I drank because I couldn't stand it any longer"). Such alibis underscore the role of cognitions in maladaptive functioning and the need for cognitive restructuring.

Cognitive restructuring process proceeds by discussing the adaptive cognitive responses that are to become part of the client's coping repertoire. The group members are taught to handle stress by substituting these alternative cognitions for the stress-engendering cognitions. The members, in other words, are instructed to "fill their minds up" with coping responses in the form of adaptive covert self-statements and/or imagery, instead of with distress-eliciting internal dialogue. The restructuring process also involves an examination of the meaning of certain A.A. slogans in the context of coping skills training. The first slogan discussed is, "Don't project." This expression is understood as the instruction not to participate in useless worry about the future. Many negative cognitive responses to stress involve irrelevant dwelling on anticipated feared events and consequences. Using this slogan to control worrisome cognitions is similar to the technique of thought stoppage discussed earlier. However, the former relates specifically to anticipated occurrences, whereas thought stoppage is more general in scope. Furthermore, the effectiveness of the instruction not to project relies on acceptance of a particular attitude or philosophy about coping that need not be present in all cases of effective thought stoppage.

A.A. counsels "Live one day at a time," i.e., to focus on what the priorities and concerns of a given day happen to be, rather than focusing on ruminative thoughts about the future. The individual may also use this maxim as a reminder to generate more useful coping behavior.

Because of an intense emotional reaction such as panic, or a deficit in the coping repertoire, a person may have difficulty imagining what to do once a negative cognition has been interrupted. When the level of emotional arousal or coping deficit interferes with generating cognitive coping procedures, the person should use the slogan, "First things first" to initiate task-guiding statements, which specify, step by step, the procedure to be followed for accomplishing some task. The individual covertly asks "What do I have to do first?" and answers in another covert self-statement (e.g., "Just begin qualifying by slowly saying your name."). When that first step is completed, the person may repeat the question ("Now, what do I have to do first?") and state what the very next step is ("Tell them about your first drink."). The task at hand is broken down into manageable steps in accordance with the A.A. slogan, "Keep it simple." Further refinements on this task-oriented approach to coping are detailed by Meichenbaum (1977) and by Meichenbaum and Goodman (1971).

In A.A. the alcoholic is told to remind him- or herself that the discomfort of remaining abstinent is not so severe that it cannot be borne for today. Each day, the individual sets the goal of remaining abstinent "just for today." The specified length of coping time may be set for very small intervals (e.g. three minutes), and can be reset as often as needed. The person is also encouraged to use the slogan, "This too shall pass" to challenge the projection that the discomfort will last forever, thereby making it easier to tolerate.

The group is taught that the coping strategies for remaining abstinent can be used to handle stress. This involves repeatedly telling oneself that the stress is bearable ("I won't be destroyed by it"), setting repeated goals to handle the stress over short periods of time, and reassuring oneself that the situation will pass. Group participants are encouraged to find and write down lists of coping statements. The statements should include realistic reassurances and reminders (e.g., "I have been through worse and survived"). The reader is referred to Meichenbaum and Turk (1976) for a list of numerous coping statements that patients can use. The patients are encouraged to practice covertly saying these statements in reassuring tones of voice.

Some people resist employing coping statements. They protest that what they anticipate happening, or what they experience, is indeed horrible, and so why shouldn't that be what they tell themselves? One way for the therapist to handle this involves examining another A.A. method for stemming the urge and rationalization for drinking—to "think a drink through." This means to think about the aversive consequences that typically follow drinking. The excuses for drinking can then be seen for what they are—bad rationalizations. The individual who defends a stress-inducing reaction to an event has failed to realize that the important issue is not the truth or falsity of the description of the event, but rather simply the prevention of unnecessary stress and the facilitation of coping skills. If doing something brings no good, then it is preferable not to do it. Hence, any reasons given in support of negative cognitions are to be viewed as rationalizations for dysfunctional behavior. To foster appreciation for this philosophy, the patients are encouraged to recall actual undesired effects to stress when their response incorporated mainly negative cognitive behavior rather than a strategy involving coping skills.

A useful way to present the philosophy of coping is through a discussion of the Serenity Prayer: "God grant me the serenity to accept the things I cannot change, courage to change the things I can, and wisdom to know the difference." Group participants can discuss why it is preferable to have serenity even when facing an unavoidable and undesirable event. Acceptance of the Serenity Prayer allows the individual to deal with a stressor via the self-instruction to "turn it over"—to cease futile preoccupation with, and craving for, what is not now, or cannot be, the case.

Coping with stressors will be enhanced if the patients are taught ways to identify when their negative appraisals distort reality. Two techniques that help people to gain some perspective on their thinking are the "so what if..." and "blow up" strategies (Lazarus, 1971). In the first, the person is requested to imagine and verbalize the presumed negative consequences of a contemplated action or event. In the second, the person is asked to deliberately exaggerate the negative consequences to the point at which they begin to seem unlikely and absurd. Both techniques allow the individual to utilize reality testing skills.

The "R" Step

The last step of S.O.B.E.R. is "R" for Recognition. This is a reminder to use self-statements that reflect cognizance of one's coping strengths and successes before ("I've been able to handle worse"), during ("I am doing Okay"), and after ("I was able to hold down the anxiety") the trigger event. In this way, the person sustains motivation to use coping skills and develops trust in his or her ability to manage stress without resorting to mood-altering drugs. This, of course, is the goal of the S.O.B.E.R. program.

REFERENCES

Beck, A.T. *Cognitive therapy and emotional disorders*. New York: International Universities Press, 1976.

Benson, H. *The relaxation response*. New York: William Morrow, 1975.

Bernstein, D.A., & Borkovec, T.D. *Progressive relaxation training*. Champaign, Ill.: Research Press, 1976.

Carrington, P. *Freedom in meditation*. New York: Anchor Books, 1978.

Criddle, W.D. The ABC theory of emotions and its application to alcoholism. *Journal of Alcohol and Drug Education*, 1977, 22(2), 4-9.

Ellis, A. *Reason and emotion in psychotherapy*. Secaucus, N.J.: Citadel Press, 1962.

Ellis, A. *Humanistic psychotherapy*. New York: McGraw-Hill, 1973.

Ellis, A., & Harper, R.A. *A new guide to rational living*. N. Hollywood, Calif.: Wilshire Book Company, 1977.

Goldfried, M.R., & Davidson, G.C. *Clinical behavior therapy*. New York: Holt, Rinehart, & Winston, 1976.

Grau, A.F. Dealing with the irrationality of alcoholic drinking. In Wolfe, J. & Brand, E. (Eds.), *Twenty years of rational therapy*. New York: Institute for Rational Living, 1977.

Higbee, J.N. RET in dealing with alcohol-dependent persons. In Wolfe, J. & Brand, E. (Eds.), *Twenty years of rational therapy*. New York: Institute for Rational Living, 1977.

Hindman, M. Rational emotive therapy in alcoholism treatment. *Alcohol Health and Research World*, 1976, 2, 13-17.

Jackson, P., & Oei, T. Social skills training and cognitive restructuring with alcoholics. *Drug and Alcohol Dependence*, 1978, 3, 369-374.

Jacobson, E. *Progressive relaxation*. Chicago: University of Chicago Press, 1929.

Lazarus, A. New techniques for behavioral change. Rational Living, 1971, 6(1). 6-7.

Mahoney, M.J. Cognition and behavior modification. Cambridge, MA: Ballinger, 1974.

May, J.R., & Johnson, J. Physiological activity to internally elicited arousal and inhibitory thoughts. *Journal of Abnormal Psychology*, 1973, 82, 239-245.

McCourt, W., & Glantz, M. Cognitive behavior therapy in groups for alcoholics. *Journal of Studies on Alcohol*. 1980, 41 (3), 338-346.

Meichenbaum, D. *Cognitive-behavior modification: An integrative approach*. New York: Plenum Press, 1977.

Meichenbaum, D., & Goodman, J. Training impulsive children to talk to themselves: A means of developing self-control. *Journal of Abnormal Psychology*, 1971, 77, 115-125.

Meichenbaum, D., & Turk, D. The cognitive-behavioral management of anxiety. In Davidson, P.O. (Ed.), *The behavioral management of anxiety, depression, and pain*. New York: Brunner/Mazel, 1976.

Novaco, R.W. Anger and coping with stress: Cognitive behavioral interventions. In Foreyt, J. & Rathjen, D. (Eds.), *Cognitive behavior therapy*. New York: Plenum Press, 1978.

Rimm, D.C. & Litvak, S.B. Self-verbalization and emotional arousal. *Journal of Abnormal Psychology*, 1969, 74, 181-187.

Rimm, D.C., & Masters, J.C. *Behavior therapy* (2nd ed.). New York: Academic Press, 1979.

Russell, P.L., & Brandsman, J.M. A theoretical and empirical integration of the rational-emotive and classical conditioning theories. *Journal of Consulting and Clinical Psychology*, 1974, 42, 389-397.

Sanchez-Craig, M. A self-control strategy for drinking tendencies. *Ontario Psychologist*, 1975, 7, 25-29.

Schachter, S. The interaction of cognitive and physiological determinants of an anxiety state. In Spielberger, C.D. (Ed.), *Anxiety and behavior*. New York: Academic Press, 1966.

Schwartz, G.E. Cardiac responses to self-induced thoughts. *Psychophysiology*, 1971, 8, 462-467.

Snyder, V. Cognitive approaches in the treatment of alcoholism. *Social Casework*. 1975, 56 (8), 480-485.

Suinn, R.M., & Richardson, F. Anxiety management training: A nonspecific behavior therapy program for anxiety control. *Behavior Therapy*, 1971, *2*, 498-510.

Velten, E.A. A laboratory task for induction of mood states. *Behavior Research and Therapy*, 1968, *6*, 473-482.

Wolpe, J. *Psychotherapy by reciprocal inhibition*. Stanford, Calif.: Stanford University Press, 1958.

ASSERTIVENESS IN RECOVERY

Sharon B. Orosz

ABSTRACT. This paper is a presentation of the theory and use of Assertiveness in Recovery groups as a model of intervention with alcoholics and significant others during the recovery phase of alcoholism. It focuses upon a rationale that many alcohol-affected individuals need specialized help in changing characteristically dysfunctional drinking behavior and suggests that assertiveness training techniques within a social groupwork format can be adapted adequately to this need.

Introduction

The treatment of alcoholism has been developing rapidly and positively over the past decade. Emphasis on the treatment of the alcoholic has been understandably focused upon achieving and maintaining sobriety. For the significant others, major attention has been upon education around alcoholism and understanding the illness as a family disease. This appears to be an appropriate beginning; however, alcoholism treatment modalities seem to lack a response to the special needs of people in the recovery phase. After all, recovery from alcoholism is a lifelong process, and specialized programs are needed to enhance the quality of sobriety.

This paper discusses the nature of the sobriety phase of recovery for both the alcoholic and significant others. Using illustrative examples, a model of intervention called Assertiveness in Recovery will be presented as a response to some of the specialized needs of the alcoholics during the recovery period.

Sobriety

Sobriety is expected to bring happy times and a bright future to both the alcoholic and significant others. Such expectations are often unrealistic, and the reality is startling and frightening.

Sharon B. Orosz, MSW, is a social worker at CNDNJ's Community Mental Health Center at Rutgers Medical School, Industrial Human Resources Unit, Piscataway, NJ.

25

The Alcoholic

The primary emotional struggle of the alcoholic in early sobriety is maintaining tight control over his or her impulses. He or she becomes emotionally flat and lacks spontaneity. Both passive and aggressive behaviors are exhibited—passivity by repression of feelings and aggression through sporadic uncontrollable outbursts (Zimberg, Wallace, & Blume, 1978). Relationships with others are stilted. It is difficult to relate to alienated family members. Handling interpersonal conflict is painful; therefore, the alcoholic minimizes or avoids it. He or she is fearful of closeness, rejection, failure, and success. Sobriety magnifies these fears.

The alcoholic and family members begin to feel for the first time that the "pink cloud" has burst. They adopt an all-or-nothing, rigid attitude and have difficulty finding a balance in life. These attitudes lead to frustration and feelings of disappointment on both sides, feelings that were apparent in the drinking state as well. Without conscious effort, sobriety does not make for positive behaviors and comfortable feelings.

The alcoholic is also subject to stresses in the external world. Everyday situations are a struggle, and often the alcoholic has only drinking behaviors in his or her repertoire. With the removal of alcohol, the individual is in a state of normlessness, often reacting to situations, particularly those which are stressful or conflictive, with familiar but unproductive behaviors.

The Significant Others

Alcoholism is a family disease; it involves and affects all family members. Plagued by unpleasant memories, they look to a problem-free future. Dulfano (Zimberg, Wallace, & Blume, 1978) suggests that alcoholic behavior is built into the family's equilibrium and does not vanish with the onset of sobriety. The once predictable drunk is no longer so predictable. Roles begin to change as children lose their adult status and spouses are asked to relinquish responsibility to the "new" family member. Individuals struggle with fears of a relapse. "Walking on eggs" becomes a common practice. The family experiences overwhelming anomie. Removal of alcoholic behavior becomes a threat to the family system, and members respond with old patterns of behavior.

Dysfunctional behavior is apparent in both the drinker and significant others in the drinking and recovery phases. For example, a low tolerance for frustration is evident in both phases. The inability to stand not having the world respond the way one wants it to, when one wants it to, is a core problem (Wolfe, 1979). Behavior change comes slowly and progresses with the length of sobriety; however, individuals must first become aware of past and present behaviors in order to make definite changes in old behavior patterns.

A.A. and Al-Anon are often primary and beginning interventions. Through A.A. and professional counseling, individuals begin to recognize and identify their feelings. Such realizations can be immobilizing, as they have trouble developing an appropriate balance in their behaviors. The tendency to focus on negative experiences from the past can impede growth and change.

Purpose, Structure, and Goals of Assertiveness in Recovery Groups

Zimberg, Wallace, and Blume (1978) set forth the premise that "successful adjustment to life without alcohol requires new responses to situations that would have prompted drinking in the past." Implicit in this statement is the need to enable alcoholics and significant others to not only examine but to change their behavior in view of their responses to tension, stress, and feelings of inadequacy, which in the past have resulted in abusive use of alcohol and dysfunctional behavior.

Assertiveness in Recovery groups attempt to actualize this theory by the use of assertive techniques in a social groupwork setting. This modality responds to the anomie that develops in the family system and other significant relationships when alcohol is removed. The group encourages the establishment of interdependence on peer members rather than dependency on one person (Zimberg, Wallace, & Blume, 1978).

The purpose of Assertiveness in Recovery groups is to focus attention on the different types of assertive behavior, as well as to improve each individual's assertiveness skills. The first four to five sessions include a variety of structured activities designed to promote a thorough understanding of the theories and procedures that are necessary for developing assertive behavior. Every effort is made to ensure that each group member develops a solid frame of reference. Structured exercises are used to cover common social situations in which assertive difficulties· frequently arise. Situations common in alcoholic families are included as illustrations.

Participants are asked to explore how their thoughts affect their feelings and behaviors, and to share these discoveries with other group members. Sharing is essential to assertiveness, as it provides group members with closeness and support at a time when they are confused and alone. Sharing of values, beliefs, and feelings allows for individual clarification. After group members are familiar with assertive terms and have expressed feelings, thoughts, and judgements, loosely structured activities are used to build assertive skills. Group members are given the opportunity to practice these skills through a behavior rehearsal technique. Behavior rehearsal is essential as it provides participants with time to experiment with their assertive behavior, to work through their fears, and to receive feedback from other participants and group leaders in a supportive, caring manner. It is hoped that group members will gain confidence and learn more about their behavior as a result of effective feedback.

Participants are asked to be aware of assertiveness issues that develop between sessions. Time is provided each session to discuss these issues. Group members are encouraged to discuss both successes and failures, ask questions, or make comments.

The last four to five sessions are devoted to the use of behavior rehearsal techniques, in which emphasis is placed on specific situations that are realistic for each participant, and that may include situations that develop with family members, friends, and/or employers. One person works on his or her personal situation at a time. These role-plays are used to help the individual gain confidence in addition to providing reinforcement to newly learned behaviors.

Length of the group varies with size and particular needs of the group participants, but averages from eight to twelve weeks, each session being at least two hours long.

Group Composition

It is recommended that Assertiveness in Recovery groups consist of no more than 12 participants, with two group leaders facilitating. Group leaders should have a brief interview with all candidates, preferably in person, to explain clearly the goals and format for the group and to question candidates about their expectations and needs (Lange & Jakubowski, 1977). Prescreening is necessary to ensure the appropriateness of participants.

Both alcoholics and significant others may be accepted to the group(s). Alcoholics should have a minimum of 90 days sobriety, but longer sobriety is desirable. Individuals experiencing dysfunctional behavior in recovery are highly suited for this group. Gaining insight into feelings is not the primary focus of the group; therefore, appropriate group members are those who have exhibited the ability to recognize and identify feelings. Individuals who appear to be invested in hanging onto unproductive behavior should be avoided. Significant others should be discouraged from participation in the same group with the alcoholic, because there may be assertiveness issues between them that need to be resolved. If both are present, there is no opportunity for rehearsal.

Leadership Issues

Group dynamics and group process are closely monitored throughout, and a high degree of competency and flexibility with the assertiveness program media is necessary. Group leaders must be sensitive to phases of group development in order to create a supportive and safe environment for members. It is essential that leaders work out a cooperative plan of facilitation. Leaders may take part in structured exercises in order to model different types of behavior. At times it may by necessary to abort the use of some structured activities, because other group needs may take priority. This program is a combination of models, and professional practitioners need to be able to adapt to the situation at hand.

The Interventive Model in Practice

Following are some illustrations of the use of assertive techniques with alcoholics and significant others in a program called "Assertiveness in Recovery" conducted at the Center for Industrial Human Resources of the Community Mental Health Center, Rutgers Medical School.

Rational-Emotive Therapy in Assertiveness

The major tenet of rational–emotive therapy is that dysfunctional emotions or behaviors are not caused by the situation but rather by what the person believes about the situation or event (Wolfe, 1979). This has particular relevance to behavior. Hence, rational–emotive therapy is a fundamental tool in assertiveness training.

One group member, related an incident that happened at work where she accidently ruined some important data. Barbara refrained from telling her boss, as her fears about the consequences were overwhelming for her. Barbara was asked to think about her irrational beliefs about the situation. She responded by saying, "He would hate me...call me names...tell everyone else in the office...take my raise away," and that this would be unbearable. She was then asked to explore the consequences of her beliefs. She realized that these beliefs caused her to avoid her boss all day, and aided in her feelings of worthlessness, self-blame, and guilt. Barbara was then asked to think of rational beliefs about the situation. Her reponse was, "Other workers have done this. I can't possibly be the only one! Everyone makes mistakes. He may understand and if he doesn't it won't be the end of the world! I'm not a terrible person just because I made a mistake." Barbara was asked to role-play the situation. She agreed, and behavior rehearsal followed, involving all the group members. Afterward, Barbara shared that her anxiety level had diminished.

I-Language Assertion

Ellen, the spouse of an active alcoholic, expressed her need to share her feelings with her husband about drinking and driving. The entire group was mobilized to the task of assisting Ellen in constructing an I-statement that adequately and sensitively delivered her message. Members were engaged in helping Ellen work through her thoughts and feelings. This statement is a result of placing these into her own style of communication: "I feel terrified when you drive after you've been drinking because I'm afraid that you'll be killed and then I'll be alone and without the man I love."

I-language assertion is particularly useful as a guide for helping people to assertively express difficult negative feelings (Lange & Jakubowski, 1977).

Group Development

The group began with the usual fears and anxieties exhibited in early phases of group development. Members also shared feelings of excitement and hope. As the group progressed, participants felt safe confronting and supporting each other. Free exchange at the beginning of each session aided in the development of group cohesion. A high degree of comfort with the behavior rehearsal technique was acquired by most participants. As expected, participants experienced feelings of sadness and loss at the time of termination. Arrangement of a follow-up session six to eight weeks after ending is often useful, as group members are in need of continued support.

Conclusion

Assertiveness In Recovery groups are easily adapted to a variety of groups. Activities and exercises can be used spontaneously in individual sessions and other types of therapy groups. This modality supports the development of the individual's human potential, recognizing that this has been inhibited for a significant period of time, during which dysfunctional behavior has been learned and firmly entrenched. It is suggested that these behaviors will persist unless a conscious and systematic process of behavior change is employed.

Support of sobriety and the identification of feelings, without assisting the individual to acquire alternate ways of responding to stressful situations, neglects an important part of the treatment process. New ways of behaving must be incorporated to improve the quality of recovery.

REFERENCES

Lange, A.J., & Jakubowski, P. *Responsible assertive behavior*. Champaign, IL: Research Press, 1977.
Wolfe, J.L. A cognitive/behavioral approach to working with women alcoholics. In Burtle, V. (Ed.), *Women who drink*. Springfield, IL: Charles C. Thomas, 1979.
Zimberg, S., Wallace, J., & Blume, S. *Practical approaches to alcoholism psychotherapy*. New York: Plenum Press, 1978.

SUGGESTED READINGS

Bailey, M.B. *Alcoholism and family casework*. New York: The Community Council of Greater New York, 1968.
Jackson, J. The adjustment of the family to the crises of alcoholism. *Quarterly Journal of Studies of Alcohol*, 1954, *15*(4), 562-586.
Klein, A.F. *Effective groupwork: An introduction to principle and method*. New York: Association Press, 1972.
Materi, M. Assertiveness training: A catalyst for behavioral change. *Alcohol Health and Research World*, 1977, Vol. I, 23-26.

A SHORT-TERM GROUP TREATMENT MODEL FOR PROBLEM-DRINKING DRIVERS

William C. Panepinto
James A. Garrett
William R. Williford
John A. Priebe

ABSTRACT. Problem-drinking drivers have, from the outset of the New York State Program in 1975, presented a real challenge to alcoholism treatment providers. The very nature of the "mandated" condition of treatment as a prerequisite for return of a driver's license lends itself to resistance and rage. A short-term group treatment model is a response to the difficulties encountered in fitting the problem-drinking driver into a treatment system that is primarily designed for latter stage-alcoholics in need of long-term, intensive rehabilitation. The short-term group approach is an application of situational crisis theory, adjustment demand theory, and treatment contracting. The intervention model begins with two individual/family evaluation sessions followed by from twelve to sixteen group therapy sessions of ninety minutes duration each.

Introduction

In 1980, outpatient alcoholism treatment agencies in New York State provided evaluation and treatment services to approximately 7000 persons referred from Drinking Driver Programs as well as to approximately 3000 persons referred from Relicensing Review Boards, both of which are programs of the New York State Department of Motor Vehicles. Convicted motorists represent about one-half of referrals to all New York State outpatient alcoholism agencies outside of New York City. This presents an excellent opportunity to intervene with a significant population that is not in the later stages of alcoholism. Clinical profiles indicate some disruption in family, work, and social relationships and the beginnings of physiological damage as evidenced by abnormal liver profiles and tissue tolerance and by alcoholic blackouts.

William C. Panepinto, CSW, is Assistant Director for Treatment and Rehabilitation; James A. Garrett, CSW, is Acting Associate Deputy Director; William R. Williford, MPH, is Assistant Director, Alcohol and Highway Safety; and John A. Priebe is Western District Director of New York State Division of Alcoholism and Alcohol Abuse, 194 Washington Avenue, Albany, NY.

Problem-drinking drivers have, from the outset of the New York State program in 1975, presented a real challenge to alcoholism treatment providers. The very nature of the "mandated" condition of treatment as a prerequisite for return of a driver's license lends itself to resistance and rage. This is compounded by the reality of the patient's current level of functioning—he or she has not usually progressed to a later stage of alcoholism. Not only does this contribute to alcoholic denial, but it also demands a different treatment response.

Treatment Approaches

A short-term group treatment model is a response to the difficulties encountered in fitting the problem-drinking driver into a treatment system which is primarily designed for latter stage alcoholics in need of long-term intensive rehabilitation. The short-term approach is an application of situational crisis theory. Social workers in various settings have long recognized the efficacy of timely intervention when a person or family is in the midst of crisis. Likewise, the impact of acute stress on a person or family already experiencing chronic stress is a well-known dynamic. The application to the problem-drinking driver target population has not yet been drawn. A second complementary theoretical construct is the "adjustment demand" model, which describes crisis problem-solving behavior as responses to task-oriented and defense-oriented adjustment demands. The third practice theory construct is treatment contracting, the mutual worker-client consensual process that defines treatment goals, tasks, and time dimensions.

Crisis theory, as classically articulated by Rapaport (1965), provides a basic conceptual framework for the treatment of problem-drinking drivers. A hazardous event, the Driving While Intoxicated (DWI) arrest, and subsequent adjudication creates for the individual a problem which he or she may view as a threat, a loss, or a challenge. The threat may be to fundamental needs or to the person's sense of ego-integrity, and it will engender varying degrees of anxiety. The loss may be actual or may be experienced as deprivation and will engender varying degrees of depression. If the problem is viewed as a challenge, it will engender a mobilization of energy.

Rapaport (1965) describes a crisis as an upset in the person's equilibrium; it may trigger old threats and conflicts, and it can't be solved by one's habitual problem-solving methods. It is time-limited, and resolution may result in either a return to the previous level of functioning or to a lower or higher level of mental health. During the crisis period, the person is more susceptible to the influence of others, and thus well-timed short-term intervention can have lasting positive effects. The following are necessary for healthy crisis resolution: (1) correct cognitive perception of the situation furthered by new knowledge; (2) management of feelings through awareness and verbalization leading to tension discharge and mastery; and (3) development of patterns of seeking and using help.

The Driving While Intoxicated (DWI) cluster of experiences, including arrest, booking, arraignment, adjudication, public notification, and referral to an alcoholism treatment agency, is indeed a situational crisis. There are clearly elements of both threat and loss present, with anxiety, depression, and anger secondary to both. It is primarily the task of the treatment staff to help the person view the crisis as a challenge, as an opportunity to resolve his or her problem drinking. Concurrently, treatment staff must cope with the person's anxiety, depression, and anger. The factors necessary for healthy crisis resolution must be present in the treatment setting. The correct cognitive perceptions and new knowledge relate to the clarity and consistency of the staff and the information provided. The management of negative feelings for tension discharge and mastery must be encouraged, supported, given structure, and not seen as a personal attack. The development of patterns of seeking and using help are dependent upon the style and content of the treatment services and the degree of trust and belief engendered. Essential to this process is the belief by treatment staff that a ''mandated'' client can make positive change. Equally important is the corollary staff belief that the intervention will have positive impact. Indeed, both client and worker must see the ''challenge'' aspects of the process.

A secondary complementary theoretical construct flows from crisis theory. The adjustment demand model describes problem-solving behavior as a response to task-oriented and defense-oriented demands as part of problem solving during a crisis. As described by Garrett (1980), the major components of stress are frustration, conflict, pressures, and overload. The frustration inherent in the DWI cluster of experiences involves loss of driver's license, sense of failure through the personalization of the experience, lack of resources to deal with the legal and treatment systems, and the delays all along the process. Conflict ranges from approach-avoidance conflicts centering on participation in alcoholism treatment to win back one's license, even if there is no self-perception of a problem, all the way to double-avoidance conflicts, experienced when losing a license or entering treatment is too threatening. The pressures and overload are legal, including arrest, imprisonment, and court experiences; fiscal, including attorney's and treatment fees, increased insurance premiums, lost wages, etc.; family pressures; and social pressures, including the public nature of disclosure.

These stresses create anxiety, depression, and anger during the crisis period. A task-oriented adjustment is the equivalent of responding to a crisis as a challenge, to develop new methods of problem-solving. A defense-oriented adjustment is the equivalent of maladaptive coping behavior in which anger, both passively and aggressively expressed, is directed at those in the helping role, and projection and suspicion are in evidence. As Panepinto and Higgins (1969) described, the clinician must "demonstrate consideration for the patient's lowered self-esteem, reduce his frustration, establish and maintain a pattern of continuity of care, and communicate interest and concern through action. An absence of controls by the therapist is poorly tolerated by and quite threatening to a patient who is leaning toward loss of ego control."

The third practice theory construct is treatment contracting, the mutual worker-client consensual process that defines treatment goals, tasks, and time dimensions. According to Seabury (1976), a treatment contract specifies the purpose of the interaction, target problems, goals and objectives, administrative procedures and constraints, roles of the participants, techniques to be used, and the time limitations of the contract. Contract stages begin with exploration and negotiation, continue through tentative agreement to the contract work phase, and end with a termination phase.

In the context of a "mandated" patient population, contracting is essential to provide clear and consistent definitions and boundaries, ground rules, and respective responsibilities. The contracting process not only provides answers to such questions as, "What do I have to do to get my driver's license back?", but also intrinsically demands participation on the part of the usually angry and reluctant patient. Contracting is problem-solving behavior; it is task-oriented adjustment demand behavior. Since treatment contracting leads to clarity and consistency, it is an excellent device in dealing with projection and suspicion. The application of contracting to a group modality, especially a short-term group intervention, is conducive to the development of a group process.

Applying DWI Characteristics to the Short-Term Group

The intervention model itself begins with two individual/family evaluation sessions, during which evaluation and treatment contracting occur. This is followed by from twelve to sixteen group therapy sessions of ninety minutes duration each. Each session focuses on drinking-driving and drinking-related treatment goals. Problem-solving alternatives are discussed, as are the kinds and depths of feelings being generated by the stressful sequence of events. The development of group identification, support, and reality questioning is encouraged. This group process represents a constructive use of coercion to confront the negative consequences of the patient's drinking behavior. Upon completion of the group experience, an individual/family session is conducted, aimed at reaching a consensus as to whether or not further treatment is indicated, and in what form and for what duration.

According to Moskowitz, Walker, and Gomberg (1979), the Driving While Intoxicated (DWI) driver is an alcohol abuser with behavioral trends that approach those of the alcoholic in treatment, although his or her drinking problems have not reached the extremes of most alcoholics in treatment (see Table 1). The DWI driver tends to have more resources, especially in terms of family relationships and steady employment, than the typical later-stage alcoholic in treatment. On most variables, the profile of the DWI driver falls between that of the control driver and the alcoholic in treatment. Personality scales that measure depression, paranoia, self-esteem, responsibility, and control of aggressive feelings show the DWI clearly between the two poles. Michigan Alcoholism Screening Test (MAST) scores show that 54 to 74 percent of DWI drivers score more than five points, which indicates problem drinking, but 99 percent of alcoholics in treatment score more than five points. In using a group modality, the presence of DWI drivers with low MAST scores will be counterproductive, contributing to group denial. Prior treatment history shows a DWI range from 2 to 42 percent, whereas alcoholics in treatment range from 50 to 71 percent. Only those DWIs with previous treatment histories would appear to be more readily able to enter the ongoing treatment system services.

Perception of drinking as a problem highlights the recent difficulties in integrating DWIs into the traditional alcoholism treatment system. The range for DWIs is 20 to 37 percent, contrasted with 81 percent of alcoholics in treatment and 3 percent of control drivers. An important strategy for group treatment formation flows from Slavson's classic technique of heterogeneous group makeup. It is critical to have several problem-drinking drivers who perceive alcohol as a problem and are verbal as members of every DWI short-term group.

The reasons given for drinking by DWI individuals show a pattern similar to that of alcoholics and can be interpreted to DWI drivers as an indicator of the progressive nature of alcohol abuse. The reasons most often cited are to ease tension, cope with personal problems, relieve fears, overcome shyness, relax, and conform to group pressure.

The cluster of variables describing problems related to drinking can also

Table 1
A Comparison of Demographic and Psychosocial Characteristics of DWI Drivers, Control Drivers, and Alcoholics in Treatment[a]

Category	Control Drivers	DWI Drivers	Alcoholics in Treatment
Divorced or separated	5-7%	22-41%	50-60%
Unemployed	4-8%	9-18%	50-60%
Blue collar occupation	42-60%	49-79%	60-80%
Income	$11,100	$9400	$9300
Self-esteem, responsibility, control of aggression[b]	Most	Intermediate	Least
Diagnosis of problem drinking (MAST)	2.46-2.61 (10% > 5)	4.22-4.77 (54-74% > 5)	6.54-6.73 (99% > 5)
Prior treatment history	0%	2-42%	50-71%
Perception of problem drinking	3%	20-37%	81%
Drink daily	10%	38%	54%[d]
Have 7 drinks at a single sitting	17%	41%	81%[e]
Drink to "cope with personal problems, ease tension, relieve fears, overcome shyness, to relax, as a habit, under group pressure"[c]	Least	Intermediate	Most
Have problems related to drinking:			
Poor health	3.9%	20%	40%
Family	2%	30%	92%[d]
Financial	0%	7%	32%[d]
Lost job	0%	7%	37%[e]
Job threatened	0%	2%	14%[d]
Quit job	0%	1%	15%[e]
Prior DWI arrests	2%	96%	56%[b]

[a]From Moskowitz, Walker, and Gomberg (1979).

[b]From Selzer, Vinoker, and Wilson (1977).

[c]From Pollack (1969).

[d]From Bell, Warheit, and Sanders (1978).

[e]From Zelhart, Schurr, and Brown (1975).

be used to demonstrate to DWI individuals that many of them have moved farther away from the control driver profile and closer to the alcoholic in treatment profile. However, this content area must be used discretely, since sweeping generalities can be counterproductive and lead to reinforcement of rationalization and denial. Family problems due to drinking are reported by 2 percent of controls, 30 percent of the DWIs, and 92 percent of the alcoholics in treatment. While 5 to 7 percent of controls are divorced or separated, 22 to 41 percent of DWIs and 50 percent of alcoholics are divorced or separated. A group discussion focusing on incipient problems as well as major problems in the family is indicated. The group should contain several members who have major family problems. Physical health status shows 4 percent of the controls reporting poor health, contrasted to 20 percent of the DWIs and 40 percent of the alcoholics in treatment. Again, focusing on early symptoms of alcohol-related health problems and eliciting such history from those in the DWI group who have already experienced health problems are indicated.

Job-related problems do not seem to be a fruitful content area for demonstrating the progression. Only 1 percent of DWIs report quitting a job due to drinking, as contrasted to 15 percent of alcoholics in treatment; only 2 percent of DWIs report threats to their job, versus 14 percent of alcoholics in treatment; only 7 percent report losing a job, versus 37 percent of alcoholics in treatment. Financial problems also seem to be minimally persuasive, since only 7 percent of DWIs, versus 32 percent of alcoholics in treatment, report inability to meet financial commitments due to spending on alcohol.

The area of drinking behaviors can be used to demonstrate progression. Whereas less than 10 percent of the control drivers report daily drinking, 38 percent of the DWIs and 54 percent of the alcoholics in treatment do. Not only can this behavior point to a trend toward dependence, but it also can break the stereotyped belief that if one doesn't drink daily, one is not alcoholic. A second aspect of drinking behavior should be discussed: 17 percent of the control drivers report consuming seven or more drinks at a sitting, but 41 percent of the DWIs and 82 percent of the alcoholics in treatment report that quantity of alcohol consumption. This data enables the group leader to introduce the important concepts of tolerance and psychomotor impairment.

The data concerning prior DWI arrests also should be content for group discussion: 2 percent of the controls, 96 percent of the DWIs, and 56 percent of the alcoholics in treatment have at least one prior DWI arrest. The repetitive nature of alcohol-abusing behavior and the difficulty in "controlling" behavior that has been proven to be stressful/harmful/dangerous/unpleasant are indicators of a significant pattern of alcohol abuse.

The above discussion of profile differences between control drivers, DWI individuals, and alcoholics in treatment, and the specific applications for short-term group treatment also provide a framework for in-service training of alcoholism treatment agency staff. The importance of the concept of progression must be emphasized. The history to date of the less than satisfactory interaction between DWIs and alcoholism treatment staff, with frustration felt on both sides, can be dramatically improved. Once again, careful selection of the members of a short-term group is essential.

REFERENCES

Bell, R., Warheit, G., & Sanders, G. An analytic comparison of persons arrested for driving while intoxicated and alcohol detoxification. In *Alcoholism: Clinical and Experimental Research*, 1978, *2*(3), 141-148.

Garrett, J. An adjustment demand: Resistance to alcoholism treatment with a DWI population. *Proceedings of the 8th International Conference on Alcohol, Drugs and Traffic Safety*, Stockholm, Sweden: 1980.

Moskowitz, H., Walker, J., & Gomberg, C. A comparison of demographic and psychosocial characteristics of DWI drivers, control drivers, and alcoholics. UCLA Alcohol Research Center of the Neuropsychiatric Institute, June 1979.

Panepinto, W., & Higgins, M. Keeping alcoholics in treatment. *Quarterly Journal of Studies on Alcohol*, 1969, *30*(2), 414-419.

Pollack, S. *Drinking driver and traffic safety project, Vol. I and II*. Los Angeles: U.S.C., 1969.

Rapaport, L. The state of crisis: Some theoretical considerations. In H. Parad (Ed.), *Crisis Intervention: Selected Readings*, FSAA, New York, 1965.

Seabury, B. The contract: Uses, abuses, and limitations. *Social Work*, January 1976, 16-20.

Selzer, M., Vinoker, A., & Wilson, T. A psychosocial comparision of drunken drivers and alcoholics. *Journal of Studies on Alcohol*, 1977, *38*(2), 1294-1312.

Zelhart, P., Schurr, B., & Brown, P. Drinking driver: Identification of high-risk alcoholics. In S. Israelstam & S. Lambert (Eds.), *Alcohol, Drugs and Traffic Safety*, Addiction Research Foundation, Toronto, 1975.

SPOUSE PARTICIPATION IN THE TREATMENT OF ALCOHOLISM: COMPLETION OF TREATMENT AND RECIDIVISM

Dan W. Edwards

ABSTRACT. A primary purpose of this study was to derive some empirical evidence as to whether involvement of spouses in the treatment process significantly affects completion of treatment and recidivism of the alcoholic. Case records of seventy patients admitted to a hospital alcohol intervention unit and their spouses comprised the total sample. The independent variable, spouse participation in three group educational sessions on alcohol as a drug and alcoholism as a progressive disease, was contrasted with completion of treatment and recidivism of the alcoholic patient. Data was also collected to determine which of the subjects participated in three or more outpatient sessions. Participation of spouses in the group work strategy derived from a developmental perspective was related to both dependent variables; however, calculations with respect to outpatient sessions failed to yield statistical significance. Data also suggested that the "spouse group" facilitated a better understanding of alcoholism as a progressive disease and alcohol as a drug, and also promoted a more hopeful outlook by alcoholics and their spouses.

As early as the 1960s, a sharp increase in public awareness and concern was evidenced over the increasing use of illegal drugs. Of all drugs abused in the United States, the National Commission on Marijuana and Drug Abuse indicated in 1973 that "alcohol dependence is without question the most serious drug problem in this country today (Government Printing Office, 1973). An increase in public awareness and professional concern was evidenced by recent public education efforts of the National Institute on Alcoholism and Alcohol Abuse (NIAAA), and the vast number of new facilities being opened throughout the nation for the specific purpose of offering specialized services to problem drinkers and their families. Whatever the actual incidence of alcohol abuse, no one can doubt the magnitude of

---

Dan W. Edwards, PhD, is an Associate Director at the School of Social Welfare, Louisiana State University.

the psychological, social, economic, and medical consequences for society. In any case, it is no wonder that social workers and other professionals are frequently confronted with the problem of alcohol abuse in all social welfare settings.

Much of the research on the treatment of alcoholism has focused primarily on the identified problem drinker. Fortunately, the role of the family in the treatment of alcoholism has begun to receive increased attention. Jackson appears to be one of the first investigators to have seriously considered the significance of the alcoholic's family in relation to alcoholism (Jackson, 1954). Nine years later, Bailey reported on alcoholism and marriage (Bailey, 1963). And in 1965, Bailey reported on Al-Anon as a resource for wives of alcoholics (Bailey, 1965). In this article, Bailey suggested that more emphasis should be placed on teaching the wives of alcoholics facts about alcoholism. One of the more notable researchers in family therapy, Jay Haley, said, "The fragmentation of the individual into parts, or the family into parts is being abandoned, and there is a growing consensus that a new ecological framework defines problems in new ways and calls for new ways in therapy" (Sager & Kaplan, 1972). The framework Haley was referring to was systems theory, which when applied to the family suggests that what affects one member of a family will also affect other members. With this in mind, the investigator interviewed all social workers who were currently working on an alcohol intervention unit. An effort was made to ascertain the most frequent concerns and problems expressed by spouses of alcoholics in the unit. The overwhelming findings were a definite lack of understanding and knowledge of alcohol as a drug and alcoholism as a disease process, as well as accompanying feelings of helplessness. It was also ascertained that only a small percentage of alcoholic patients admitted to the unit followed through with outpatient counseling after discharge, and the dropout rate before completion of treatment in the unit was considered high. Therefore, the primary purpose of this study was to derive some empirical evidence as to whether involvement of spouses of alcoholics in a group work intervention strategy significantly affects completion of treatment and recidivism of the alcoholic. An effort was also made to evaluate the expectiveness of the group.

It was assumed that a group work intervention strategy designed to provide spouses with information about alcohol as a drug and alcoholism as a disease process as well as to create an atmosphere that would facilitate mutual support, would tend to enchance social functioning of group members. It logically follows that if the social functioning of group members was enhanced, this would carry over into their relationships with their alcoholic spouses and contribute to a mutual feeling of hopefulness rather than helplessness, which was another purpose of this study.

The group work intervention strategy was based upon the developmental approach, which emphasizes social functioning rather than viewing people as problems. Further, the developmental approach suggests that everyone is confronted with troublesome developmental stages, crises and stresses with which they must cope (Falck, 1967). "More specifically, it sees people in terms of the extent to which they are realizing their potential for (1) self-awareness, self-evaluation, and self-activation; (2) awareness of individual others, valuation of others, and interaction with others, and (3) awareness of the group situation, valuation of that situation, and action through the group" (Tropp, 1977, pp. 1322–1323.

The Agency

The Alcohol Counseling Center is a large, private, nonprofit agency located in northwest Florida. Funding is derived from an eight-year staffing grant through NIAAA, and state and local matching funds, including fees charged on a sliding scale basis. The annual budget amounts to slightly more than $1,200,000 and employs approximately 150 professionals and paraprofessionals.

Services are offered through seven basic components: (1) outpatient and emergency services; (2) evening and weekend services; (3) community, outreach, industrial, and occupational services; (4) DWI (driving while intoxicated/impaired) Alcohol Education Program; (5) a 36-bed, coeducational halfway house; (6) a 20-bed, low-medical detoxification program; and (7) a 20-bed alcohol intervention unit housed in a hospital. All services are organized around a systems frame of reference, with outpatient and emergency services providing linkage with all other services. That is, every client who enters the system is assigned an outpatient counselor who is responsible for following and coordinating the client system as he or she moves through any other services that become necessary and appropriate. It should also be mentioned that the outpatient counselor is responsible for the provision of all follow-up services. Two outpatient social workers led the spouse group discussed in this investigation.

Methodology

Case records of seventy patients admitted to the hospital alcohol intervention unit in northwestern Florida and their spouses comprised the total sample. No specific method of randomization was utilized, as the first seventy married patients admitted during the four month period were selected for the study.

The sample was divided into twenty two patients and their spouses (these spouses did not participate in treatment); twenty-four patients and their spouses (these spouses participated in 1 to 2 sessions); and twenty-four patients and their spouses (these spouses participated in three or more sessions). The amount of participation of spouses in the group strategy was correlated with two dependent variables: (1) completion of treatment by diagnosed alcoholics; and (2) recidivism. The family-oriented spouse group consisted of three sessions focused on providing factual information about alcohol as a drug and alcoholism as a progressive disease, while at the same time facilitating a group atmosphere of mutual support among the spouses participating in the group.

Information about alcohol and alcoholism was presented in a didactic manner, with the social group workers encouraging interaction and mutual support among participants. Also, any information shared by group participants that did not have a factual basis was responded to by providing factual information. It was encouraging to find that the spouses were quick to form a sense of cohesiveness and readily offered mutual support. It was also interesting to note that group members were quick to empathize with each other but were also eager to explore and share thoughts and suggestions for coping with their alcoholic spouses. This was followed by two to three social casework sessions with the alcoholic and spouse, focused on preparing both for the alcoholic's return to the family and community. The sessions included the development of a contract for outpatient counseling and support. The two dependent variables were operationally defined as follows: (1) recidivism—any patient who was readmitted to the intervention unit within twelve months following discharge or release was considered a recidivist; and (2) completion of treatment—any patient who was released from the unit on an AMA (against medical advice) basis was considered as not having completed treatment. Data were also collected to determine which of the subjects participated in three or more outpatient treatment sessions and to determine the effectivenesss of the spouse group.

Subjects in all three groups failed to differ significantly in age, education, income, number of marriages, or number of children. However, spouses who elected to not participate in any of the sessions were considerably more frequently not the first legal spouse of the patient. It should also be reported that of the total subjects, only 9 percent were black; all others were white. The chi square statistical model was utilized to determine the probability that the observed distribution could not have occurred by random sampling from the expected distribution. The phi coefficient was used to calculate correlation between the alcoholics and their spouses regarding effectiveness of the group.

Findings

The data on recidivism and completion of treatment are depicted in Table 1.

Based upon the levels of significance, one might safely conclude that the observed distribution probably did not occur as a result of random sampling from the expected distribution. More specifically, it would appear that participation by spouse in a group work strategy (independent variable) is related to both dependent variables. Thirty nine of the total sample participated in three or more outpatient treatment sessions. Although all calculations with respect to outpatient sessions failed to yield statistical significance, it was interesting to note that a few more of the patients whose spouses participated in 1 to 2 sessions continued with 3 or more outpatient sessions, and a greater difference occurred between those with no spouse participation and those whose spouse participated in 3 or more sessions. That is, although this result was not statistically significant, one can conclude that, in this sample, the greater amount of spouse participation in the group, the more patients participated in 3 or more outpatient sessions.

Data in Table 2 represent an effort to evaluate the effectiveness of the group work strategy. It should be pointed out that spouses who did not participate in the group were excluded from these calculations.

The data show a perfect correlation between alcoholics' and their spouses' feelings that the group intervention strategy helped spouses to better understand alcoholism as a disease process and alcohol as a drug. The data also

Table 1
Spouse Participation Contrasted by Treatment
Completion and Recidivism

Sessions Attended	Treatment Completed*		Recidivism+	
	Yes	No	Yes	No
None	6	16	12	10
1 to 2	12	12	7	17
3 or more	18	6	7	17

*$x^2 = 10.51$, $p < .01$.
+$x^2 = 7.47$, $p < .05$.

Table 2
Educational Effectiveness of Group

Response to Question	Spouse	Alcoholic*

Do you feel the spouse group helped you (or your spouse if not a participant) better understand alcoholism as a disease and alcohol as a drug?

	Spouse	Alcoholic
Yes	48	48
No	0	0
Total	48	48

Do you feel the spouse group helped you (or your spouse if not a participant) develop a more hopeful outlook?+

	Spouse	Alcoholic
Yes	47	46
No	1	2
Total	48	48

*The correlation between spouses who participated in the group and their alcoholic spouses is .00.
+The correlation between spouses who participated in the group and their alcoholic spouses is .14.

indicate a strong correlation between alcoholics' and their spouses' feelings that participation in the group work strategy contributed to a more hopeful outlook. This strong agreement between alcoholics and their spouses would also tend to support an earlier assumption that benefits derived from the spouse group did carry over into their relationship with their alcoholic spouse(s).

Implications for Group Work Practice and Research

Given the relatively small sample and the levels of significance, the findings are very encouraging. This is particularly so when treatment personnel are able to involve the spouses of alcoholic clients in a social group strategy. Findings also serve to reify the importance of attempting to actively enlist the participation of spouses of alcoholics in treatment to further enhance the probability of the client completing treatment and to reduce the probability of recidivism. It may well be that involvement in the treatment process, coupled with information about alcohol as a drug and alcoholism as a progressive disease, may instill a sense of hopefulness rather than helplessness in the spouse, who may reinforce the same sense of hopefulness in the alcoholic.

Future studies with larger samples and samples that are representative of different sections of the country would be helpful. Further investigation is also needed to identify other possible variables that may be significantly related to alcoholic clients completing treatment, both on an inpatient and an outpatient basis. Finally, it would appear that the use of group work based upon the developmental approach—providing factual information about alcohol as a drug and alcoholism as a disease process, and promoting a group atmosphere of mutual support—does at least tentatively appear to be a worthwhile interventive measure. From a theoretical point of view, it can be assumed that spouses of alcoholics admitted for inpatient treatment do appear to be experiencing a developmental crisis. Thus, a group work strategy based upon the developmental approach can enhance the social functioning of spouses and possibly lead to a reduction in recidivism and greater likelihood of both spouse and alcoholic following through with outpatient treatment.

More specifically, in relation to social group work practice, it is clear that group methods employed in alcohol counseling centers still tend to follow fairly traditional lines, which view the client system as suffering from a problem rather than a developmental crisis. The results of this pilot investigation offer some empirical evidence that the practice of social group work from a developmental perspective is an important consideration when designing and/or selecting a particular group work strategy for the treatment of alcoholism. Findings also suggest that providing factual information to the spouses of alcoholics reduces unwarranted fear and confusion, and facilitates movement through the crisis brought about when the alcoholic is hospitalized for treatment of alcoholism.

REFERENCES

Bailey, M. B. Research on alcoholism and marriage. *Social Work Practice*. New York: Columbia University Press, 1963, pp. 19–30.

Bailey, M. B. Al-Anon family groups as an aid to wives of alcoholics. *Social Work, 10*(1), 1965, 68–74.

Falck, H. S. Crisis theory and social group work. Paper presented at the NASW Mid-Continent Regional Institute, Topeka, Kansas, November, 1967.

Government Printing Office. Drug use in America: Problem in perspective. Washington, D.C.,
    Second Report of the National Commission on Marijuana and Drug Abuse, 1973, p. 143.
Jackson, J. K. The adjustment of the family to the crises of alcoholism. *Quarterly Journal
    of Studies on Alcohol,* 1954, *24*(2), pp. 227-238.
Sager, C. J. & Kaplan, H. S. *Progress in group and family therapy.* New York: Brunner/Mazel,
    1972.
Tropp, E. Social group work: The developmental approach. *Encyclopedia of Social Work,*
    1977, *2*, pp. 1322-1323.

FOUR PLUS FOUR:
A SHORT-TERM FAMILY GROUP
FOR RELATIVES OF ALCOHOLICS

Susan Balis
Edith Zirpoli

ABSTRACT. This article describes a family group with a changing, heterogeneous, short-term membership. The host setting is an alcoholism treatment unit within a traditional, private psychiatric hospital. Family group members come on behalf of another, not for themselves. This paper treats issues of selection process, structure, objectives, themes, specific problems of this type of group, leaders' techniques for dealing with such problems, and cotherapy roles and interactions, recording both individual and group change and applicability to other settings.

What can you do within families in only 28 days of rehabilitation? The Strecker Program for the Treatment of Alcoholism offers a family group as one of the components of a diversified program. In brief, our facility for alcoholics and other substance abusers is a specialized service within an established, private psychiatric hospital in an Eastern metropolis. Our service is young—about eight years old. Each of our 26 patients has a private attending psychiatrist and participates in intensive rehabilitation comprising daily education hours, a variety of group experiences, psychotherapy, men's or women's group, community meetings, and activities therapy.

Family involvement is emphasized from the point of admission. The Family Program includes once-a-week transition group for inpatients, family members, and those recently discharged. These groups are led by a nurse and a volunteer, who is a recovering alcoholic. The transition group follows a family dinner, in turn preceded by family group, which is open to relatives and friends but not to patients. On another evening a family education

Susan Balis, MSS, and Edith Zirpoli, MSW, are social workers in the Strecker Program for the treatment of Alcoholism, The Institute, Pennsylvania Hospital, Philadelphia, PA 19139.

hour is led in rotation by a psychiatrist, nurse, psychologist, addiction counselor, and social worker. Following the education experience, families may attend Al-Anon while patients go to A.A. On Sundays, there is another Al-Anon meeting available in the afternoon, an education hour and open A.A. meeting with patients in the evening. In addition to these group experiences available to all, relatives are offered family and/or marital therapy or individual counseling. Preventive intervention for youngsters is also presented in the form of film and discussion. Thus, the family group is one among numerous components of a diversified schedule.

Composition and Criteria for Selection

Family group meets weekly for 1½ hours and is open to family and friends of the alcoholics and drug abusers. It is available during the patient's hospital stay, which is usually 4 to 6 weeks, plus four sessions postdischarge. Typically, group is attended by a dozen or so members representing seven or eight patients. Age may range from younger than sixteen to older than sixty. Meetings include parents, in-laws, spouses, siblings, and friends. For some members, this may not be their first experience with getting help: they come with a sense of failure, and the group may rekindle realistic hope.

Currently the group is led by two white female graduate social workers although leadership has been interdisciplinary, interracial and "intersexual." The only criterion for inclusion in family group is self-selection. Geography limits regular attendance, since about 25 percent of the members live hundreds of miles from our hospital, and work schedules may also impose constraints. Anger, bitterness, and estrangement thin the potential ranks initially. Often a few weeks separation will provide sufficient respite for families to recommit themselves to the recovery process and become engaged.

Probably the group experience itself has the most beneficial impact on the family members. It is unfortunately all too common that, as the addiction progresses, they become isolated from support systems. In attempts to hide the problem they often drop out of much-needed social activities. For numerous reasons they are unwilling to tell even close relatives or friends what is happening. They wind up having no outlet for their feelings and no information from others.

It is easier to be open with those who have had similar experiences and who therefore will not judge or look down on them. Members feel less guilty over their anger and ineffectiveness, and share the relief that their loved one is finally in a hospital.

Objectives

Keeping in mind that Family Group is a time-limited experience of an early stage of recovery, we limit our objectives. Recovery for the family member, just as for the alcoholic, is a slow process that must be continued well beyond this initial treatment. Goals of the family group, therefore, are to educate the members to the concept of a family illness, to allow them to identify and express their feelings and shift their focus from the addicted person to themselves, to examine their own contributions to the progression of the illness and to share with others who are going through the same experience.

As each new member enters the group, we begin with the premise that the difficulties he or she is experiencing may arise from a lack of education about the disease concept. Woven into the discussion is information on some of the phenomena that occur: enabling, overprotectiveness, trying to take responsibility for the addiction onto themselves, the availability of such resources as Al-Anon, family therapy, and individual counseling. Education, which is nonjudgmental, helps to relieve guilt, lowers defensiveness, and enables members to develop a structure for their own recovery. The very act of gaining knowledge and accepting the disease often brings a sense of mastery and subsequent ego enhancement. Another objective of group is ventilation. Families come to us depressed, frustrated, angry, guilt-ridden, and isolated. Some are still denying or minimizing the impact of the addiction on their lives. Within the immediate family, communication may have degenerated into an endless series of disagreements and misdirected expressions of anger, resentment, blame, and scapegoating of the addicted person or some other vulnerable family member. Rarely are family members able to offer each other the support and understanding they so desperately need. By the time relatives arrive at Strecker, it has often become too threatening for them to talk openly. They fear that communication of feelings will impede recovery. In family group, where the patient is not present and where members can hear the expression of negative affects, they can begin to ventilate in a supportive, nonjudgmental environment.

Prior to treatment, families have been directing virtually all their attention to the alcoholic. Family functioning has shifted to accommodate the vicissitudes of the addiction and highly charged emotions are focused around the addict. "I feel good when he is up and I feel terrible when he is down," is a statement we hear frequently. It is a difficult but essential task to shift this focus back to the relative. If the entire family is to engage in a process of recovery, it is imperative that each member begin to "own" his or her feelings. If some detachment can be achieved, then each family member will be able to move toward more autonomous functioning.

As group members can focus on themselves and work through some of their own reactions to the addiction, it may become possible for them to examine their own role in the illness. They may have unwittingly contributed to the progression of the disease; for example, the wife who calls her alcoholic husband's boss to make excuses for absences in an effort to keep him from losing his job, or the father who pays car repair bills incurred as a result of his daughter's night on the town. Families need to look at whether they may have become martyrs, enablers, or rescuers, and then must go on to take the difficult, painful steps necessary to move out of these counterproductive roles. They need to let go of their anger and guilt, attend to their own needs, build support systems for themselves, and recognize that they too are recovering from an illness. They must make plans for their continued recovery after the time in family group has ended.

Themes

It is striking how consistently certain themes present themselves over time in family group. One of the first issues a new member may be able to talk about is guilt. Whether the member is a parent, spouse, child, sibling, or even a close friend, the expressions are very similar. "If I had been more patient or understanding . . ." "If I had known that . . ." "If I had responded differently . . ." inferring or stating that the disease would have been arrested earlier. Younger children may attribute the alcoholism to their own poor school performance or misbehavior. Adult children or siblings may feel they "deserted" the alcoholic when they moved away from home or shifted involvement to their own nuclear family. Parents may assume that the addiciton is a reflection of inadequate parenting. Spouses may point to their own personal short comings or to marital conflict as the source of the illness. For some group members, guilt is an issue they've been struggling with openly for a long time before they came to us. For others, guilt has been subconscious and surfaces only gradually. The presence of guilty feelings is often indicated by denial. "I know it's not my fault" alerts us to further explore the issue of guilt.

Feelings of anger may enable the family members to avoid awareness of guilt. Anger is probably the most frequently expressed emotion for a newcomer. Defense against guilt is only one of the many probable sources of anger. It may be a reaction to the growing sense of their own powerlessness and frustration. There is anger at the impact the addiction has had on their lives. The adverse effects of shouldering more responsibility for management of the home, financial instability, conflicts with legal authorities, and attempts to cover up lead to growing social isolation. Some members of our group have an alcoholic in their family of origin and are re-experiencing unresolved anger at an earlier situation. In addition, it is not uncommon for them to feel that if the alcoholic truly loved them, he or she wouldn't be drinking. Anger often presents as a reaction to feeling hurt and worthless.

Issues of control operate on many levels. Families come to us feeling that their lives are out of control. The usual working out of who takes responsibility for what within the home may have gone unresolved for years, as all efforts were focused on a power struggle over the addiction. This can leave the family unprepared to develop or rediscover constructive techniques of problem solving and conflict resolution. Resentment may lead to overt or covert battles that involve money, sex, discipline of children or relations with the extended family. If the core issues remain undefined, these issues contaminate recovery. Family members may be unwilling or unable to let go of the power struggle and will attempt to control rehabilitation. They shift only with great difficulty to an exploration of themselves and the changes they need to make for their own recovery. An issue that contributes to the difficulty of this shift is mistrust. Intellectually, relatives may know they have to rebuild trust in the alcoholic, but there are strong pressures against it. Repeated hurt and disappointment over broken promises, lying, or abortive attempts to control drinking may have caused a family member to build a self-protective wall of cynicism and futility. It seems too painful or frightening to trust and take the risk of once again being disappointed.

One of the objectives for a successful family recovery is detachment. However, overinvolvement may preclude members from becoming aware of this concept on their own. Often group leaders must introduce the idea of "detachment with love." This is a theme relatives will hear often repeated in Al-Anon but which they may frequently misinterpret. They must learn to detach from the illness but not from the person. They must comfortably accept that control of the alcoholism belongs to the alcoholic. Families can be responsible only for their own recovery, which is different from the alcoholic's. They must understand that they are powerless over the illness but that they do have control over how they respond to it.

Complicating Factors and Solutions

Our particular type of open-ended yet short-term group poses complications, as does the heterogenous, intergenerational population. Attendance can swing from four to twenty-four but is pretty consistently a baker's dozen representing about eight families. As leaders, we have tried to capitalize on the heterogeneity and to use the members themselves to instill group norms and values. A somewhat similar self-help experience awaits them in Al-Anon or Families Anonymous. The family group can serve as preparation for such on-going fellowship associations.

At the beginning of any meeting where there are new members—the great majority of sessions—the leaders introduce themselves and ask each person to introduce him or herself and state their relationship to the patient. One or the other of us will ask if a member would like to tell the new members how the group works and what it's all about. Someone often volunteers and usually says something like, "Group is for us, not the patients. It's a place for us to talk about how we feel." If such an "auxiliary leader" does not speak to the issue of confidentiality, a leader will remind members that they want to feel comfortable in saying what's really on their minds without worrying about loss of privacy, and that they are invited to attend once a week while the patient is in the hospital and four times afterwards. We try to establish a tradition of regular attendance. At the end of the meeting the leaders ask who will not be attending the next week and request members to let them know if they should, in the interim, find themselves unable to come. Leaders try to serve as models, announcing ahead of time if one must be away and requesting permission in advance if there are to be guests. However, a firm tradition of responsibility for attendance has not been as successful as had been hoped.

Cotherapy

Cotherapy in a group with changing membership has its strains. One leader has been with a particular group for months and found the shifting composition bewildering. While members changed, the themes remained the same. Time to talk frankly with fellow leaders was helpful. There have been points in the group's history when leadership was by triumvirate rather than duo. Both felt a real sense of loss when a fellow leader recently moved to a different shift leaving only two female social workers. In spite of being the same sex and same profession, these two provide differences in age, outlook, and style. One tends to focus more on the individual and on feelings, the other on group interactions and on coping behaviors.

The leaders may have different contacts with members outside of group. One may be involved in weekly, individual meetings with a wife, while the other might be seeing a couple in marital counseling. Leaders can complement each other here: if one is supporting a dependent young wife in individual sessions, the other may confront her in group. The leaders share common objectives, and their knowledge about the themes most vital in the earlier stages of recovery is a decisive factor in keeping interventions complementary.

The leaders evolved a reasonable, not overly time-consuming method for reviewing group progress. The day after group, they meet for half an hour to exchange impressions of overall functioning and information about members. Since each leader is responsible for serving as "family person" for half of the twenty-six bed patient community, they need to clue each other in about members. They alternate responsibility for recording the group as a whole, though each takes charge of making a brief note weekly in the patient's chart.

Recording

A simple system of recording family group has evolved. It tracks four variables: leaders, members present, their relationship to the patient, and major themes. Group process, membership roles, degree of verbalization, self-revelation, expression of affect, and other important factors are not formally recorded in these notes. They may be communicated verbally or noted in the patient's chart. These brief notes yielded a consistent record stretching back to 1977 and permit comparisons over time. These records have been used to track increasing family participation in the program from its inception to the present. They help predict periodic dips in attendance and have the potential for correlating family involvement during hospitalization with patient adjustment after discharge.

Applicability

This type of short-term, open-ended family group may be applicable to a variety of settings, e.g., general and pediatric hospitals, psychiatric facilities, and specialized schools. Such settings share some of the same challenges such as shifting heterogeneous populations and the fact that family members come on behalf of another, are sensitive to issues of blaming, and initially may resist shifting their locus of attention to themselves. The rewards of such a group in terms of leaders' and members' satisfaction.

WOMEN IN GROUPS:
A PRE-GROUP EXPERIENCE FOR WOMEN
IN RECOVERY FROM ALCOHOLISM
AND OTHER ADDICTIONS

Carol Joyce
Paula Hazelton

ABSTRACT. The authors describe the development of a short-term group for women in recovery from alcoholism and other addictive patterns. This group adds a special dimension to the treatment of women. The article outlines how the group assists women in identifying goals and competencies needed to restructure their emotional and social lives.

Introduction

Sex sterotypical behavior has long been common for women, including women in recovery from addiction to alcohol and other drugs. This paper will focus on aspects of treating women in recovery in same-sex groups. These groups are seen as essential if women are to fully participate in group psychotherapy with men. Women seem to need this group, either alone, or as an adjunctive approach to be used during the early process of recovery. Group therapy offers women a laboratory for testing new behaviors within the safety of a therapeutic setting. Group also makes it possible for women to identify with other women's strengths and vulnerabilities.

The Groups

This paper reflects experience with two women's groups, each composed of five to eight women, the majority of whom were recovering alcoholics, sober a minimum of three months. The groups also had women who were

---

Carol Joyce, MA, RN, is Associate Director of BJM Center for After-Care, New York, NY. Paula Hazelton, CSW, is a Doctoral student at Columbia University, New York, NY.

non-alcoholics but whose relationships were marked by strong attachments to parents or lovers who were addicts. The groups extend eighteen sessions. They were conducted by two women, one a nurse clinical specialist and the other a social work intern interested in a group training experience. The members had little or no prior group experience and, for the most part, had come from relatively isolated lifestyles. They ranged in age from 21 to 62. Several were married and had children. Others were single professional women, some with affective disorders. They had previously been treated in psychiatric settings and then referred to alcoholism treatment. They were an interesting mix of age, work experience, family life history, as well as addictive behavior. The presence of non-alcoholic women helped members to identify with each other on various levels more quickly than in exclusively alcoholic groups, where there is a tendency to isolate alcoholism as "the" common denominator. This diffuseness seemed to have the added effect of reducing the stigma of the female alcoholic.

Role of Therapist and Cotherapist/Intern

The role of the therapists was, in keeping with traditional practice, to facilitate the resolution of group and interpersonal conflict and to act as transference figures and role models. In the groups under discussion, role modeling was of particular importance and served a dual purpose. Therapists are seen as authority figures and, as such, possess at least some "power" and leadership. Through the structured exercises, group members were encouraged to share in the power and leadership functions, which allowed them to experiment with these functions. Although initially uncomfortable with the sense of equality and inherent responsibility, most members of the group became willing to expose their strengths and abilities.

The therapist-intern relationship exemplified a supportive relationship between women. The idea of a "mentor"—particularly a female—just has not occurred to many women. The modeling of this type of relationship between women was a consciousness-raising experience. Therapist and intern modeled alternative behaviors and attitudes between themselves and in their interactions with group members. They provided "permission" for the women to explore and experiment with alternative behaviors and attitudes.

The focus of the small-group experience for women was support and early insight. Members used this experience to collectively identify strengths and goals (both as individuals and as a group), and to examine various life roles. Traditional female roles, as well as newly emerging lifestyles and nontraditional roles for women, were explored, together with the feelings and conflicts associated with each.

Alonso (1979) noted that ''women for better or worse, have developed certain specific ways of viewing and coping with the world, of managing their self-esteem and expressing their creativity. On the less positive side they have also developed a set of maladaptive defenses and behaviors that exert a negative influence on themselves and their environment.'' At the beginning in both groups, the women were self-deprecating in their comments about themselves, adamantly defending self-perceptions of weakness and dependency. There was a real pull toward dependency. Members of both groups indulged in a good deal of injustice collecting, as well as competing for the role of the sickest. The therapist, pointed out that all the women had survived very hard circumstances and managed to cope admirably. Most were actively seeking help in handling the conflicts in their lives. It seemed that there was more of a need to convince each other that they were needy, dependent and ill, than to expose common problems and share common strengths. Whenever the women's reluctance to own their real strengths was pointed out, the intervention was greeted with explosive laughter, followed by a sense of relief. They no longer needed to pretend that they were incapable or incompetent. They indeed might have felt dependent and inadequate, but all of them had somehow managed to survive financially and to some extent socially.

Group Structure and Themes

The therapists were instrumental in establishing group norms and values that would not limit or influence its female members to adhere to stereotypic feminine roles and behaviors (i.e, emotionally passive, dependent, submissive, powerless). Structured exercises, modeling, and rotating of leadership roles provided heightened awareness and opportunities for experimentation with alternative behaviors. Communication exercises, which focused on listening, feedback, and self-exposure, were devised. This reduced some of the overwhelming anxiety some of the women seemed to experience in group. A clinical example follows.

Two women were selected to sit facing each other in the center of the group. One was given a task such as: ''Tell Georgia how it feels to be in an all-women's group. Give her the positive and negative feelings. Try to be as honest as you can. Maintain eye contact.'' The instructions to the other woman were: ''Georgia, you are to listen, not to respond until Jan is finished. Then feed back to her what she said and any feelings you picked up.'' The task of the other group members was to focus on *how* the pair communicated and then to comment on the process and their feelings about the topic.

This exercise was taught with a return demonstration incorporated into the format. Group members were delighted to have the group leader and intern practice the communication exercise. One member would give the instructions and announce the topic to be discussed. She would also lead the other members in observing how well the coleaders shared their feelings and fulfilled the task they had previously taught and implemented with each of the women in the group. They were on the ''hot seat'' now—the exclusive focus of attention. In keeping with the values encouraged in the group, the therapists revealed to the members their concerns about group leadership, modeling openness, and a sense of trust and support. Wong (1976) suggested that some people find it easier to make a transition from stereotypical roles to nonstereotypical roles if they can observe a therapist of the same sex who models the nonstereotypical behavior. The leaders participated actively in all the exercises, revealing themselves, as did the group members. In this sense, the group functioned as a consciousness-raising experience.

Another essential element in fostering the understanding of the group and the active participation of the women was the use of written process recordings, as suggested by Brown and Yalom (1977). The leaders did the first few, and then the group members rotated responsibility for observing the process in the group. These written reports, which the women would bring back the following week, became an important aspect of the group members' active style of participation in the teaching process. In addition, it brought to light the hidden talents of several of the women. One young professional read people so well and wrote of her observations with such clarity and feeling that it renewed her interest in writing and poetry, for which she had a gift. Her sharing of some of her poetry and journal of feelings endeared her to the group members. Their response also encouraged her to think of returning to college. The observations in the process recordings were valued and debated. Through focusing on communications skills, learning how to observe and record interactions, and role modeling, the group was attempting to develop active, goal-oriented women who were aware of their impact on the environment.

Both alcoholic and non-alcoholic women in the group expressed anxiety and conflicting feelings about exploring ''uncharted territory.'' They simultaneously feared and felt challenged by the opportunity to strive toward individual goals, which promised to meet their own needs and to allow them to develop a sense of individuality. Frequently, alcoholic women tend to see all their problems and strivings as related exclusively to their problems with sobriety, as they previously related them to their problem with alcohol, rather than seeing them for what they are—universal problems shared by most women.

One method of looking at the issues in the lives of women used in the groups was the focus on the "critical periods" of women's lives which Maggie Scarf outlines in *Unfinished Business* (1980). Universal phases of development such as adolescence brought up rich common themes. All of the women, without exception, failed to achieve specific goals they had desired during the adolescent period. Significantly, these women, having received inadequate nurturing during their childhoods, became involved during their adolescence in caring for others. Most wanted to go to college, and some were able to achieve this goal; they had hoped that this choice would gain them freedom from the family. Many experienced the death or loss of a significant person or a move from their childhood home at this time, which was followed by depression.

Few mentioned having a sense of their own sexuality during this critical period. Most said that they were socially isolated, without friends or group activities during their adolescence. Most did not seem to know that an alternative to concealing their fears and hopes existed. Several had become artists but lived isolated lives. No one had shown these women how to go about forming relationships *outside the family*; they had no communication skills. Alternatives to the socially approved nurturing role *within the family* were lacking. As the group members became more trusting of each other, questions arose concerning the need to learn to nurture oneself and to give oneself permission to do so.

Another significant issue, which arose after some trust was established, was that of conflict between mothers and daughters. It arose in the guise of anger between two group members: Joan, at age 23 the youngest, and Martha, one of the older group members at 46, who was also a mother. Joan was perceived by Martha as pushy and demanding. Martha was perceived by Joan as being "whiny and complaining." Conflicts centering on aggression and dependency were apparent in the tension between the two. Joan had a mother who had been ill of cancer for ten years prior to Joan's entering the group. Martha had a daughter close to Joan's age. Martha had been drinking and ill during her daughter's growing years. She had now been sober four years.

Transference was dealt with by means of a structured communication exercise between the two women, in which role reversal was incorporated. The conflict and rage associated with the change in both Joan and Martha was acted out within the security of the group. The perceptions of the other group members assisted both Joan and Martha in realizing the tremendous guilt and fear they now associated to other women. Interestingly, both of these women related easily, albeit seductively, to men. The fact that the group was limited to women was important, because a group that would have included men would have distracted Joan and Martha into flirting with the men and not dealing with the issue of their dependency needs.

Both Joan and Martha were in continual conflict with other women, perceiving them as incompetent and needy. Yet, because both were actively attempting to change their lifestyle of drinking and illness into a more productive and active pursuit of their own goals, both were willing to explore their distortions about other women. Their perceptions brought up the issue of mother-daughter relationships and the problem of separation. In the context of the conflict between Joan and Martha, one member who earlier had been unable to talk about her mother became increasingly able to explore some of her angry feelings toward her mother and women in general.

Discussion

Short-term groups with women in recovery, either from alcoholism or other addictive patterns, can be valuable preparatory experience for women entering into treatment settings. Such a group is designed to be short-term (3 to 4 months). The group functions in several ways: (1) It is adjunctive treatment for women in individual therapy. (2) Frequently, it brings to the fore quickly the conflicts hidden beneath the women's strong dependency needs, which, in long-term therapy, might be explored interminably. Groups with other women, expecially women in recovery, foster more immediate recognition of the common defenses and sex role expectations that women have used to survive in this society. (3) The group functions as an educative process. It gives women concrete means of increasing their communication skills, and provides role models from literature and life, from whom they can learn the specifics of "how" to live. It seems important in the addictive process that one focus more on the "how" than the "why" of the behavior, at least initially. This also appears true for women in same-sex groups. The "how" explores the route to recovery, as well as some of the common elements of how women have arrived at this point. Exploration of the commonalities increases self-esteem, as well as offering women a handle for more assertive behaviors. The active participation of the group leaders also reduces the powerlessness that women seem to sense when they assess female authority.

Focusing on competent women and how they exercise their skills is a factor in making these groups successful. Women in mixed groups, particularly those in early sobriety, are less likely to note their competencies in the presence of men. They tend to focus on their dependency needs, fitting into the sex-role expectations of men, and behaviors are tested less easily.

This type of group is best treated as an early "pre-group" experience, or as a necessary educative and supportive process that encourages active participation and outlines more quickly the goals and competencies a woman might need in restructuring her emotional and social life.

Members of the groups were asked to summarize their experience and identify what they considered to be the most important aspect of the group. The consensus was that women were quite adept at giving, but that they needed experience and support in learning to take for themselves. The women's group offered the opportunity to be given to without having to assume a dependent and/or sick role in return.

REFERENCES

Alonso, A. Women in group therapy. *International Journal of Group Psychotherapy*, 1979, *29*, 481-491

Brown, S., & Yalom, I. D. International group therapy with alcoholics. *Journal of Studies on Alcohol*, 1977, *38*, 426-456.

Scarf, M. *Unfinished business: Pressure points in the lives of women*. New York: Doubleday, 1980.

Wong, M. R., Dazey, J., & Conrow, Ray M. Expanding masculinity: Counseling the male in transition. *Counseling Psychology*, 1976, *6*, 58-60.

GROUP TREATMENT OF CHILDREN FROM ALCOHOLIC FAMILIES

Kendra-Ann Brown
Jeffrey Sunshine

ABSTRACT. Children from alcoholic families comprise a vulnerable population whose lives can be changed significantly through appropriate intervention. This fact is even more important in light of recent evidence that children from alcoholic homes have a high incidence of alcoholism as adults (Black, 1981). Groups can be an effective method of providing intervention. Alcoholism often damages relationships, and groups provide an opportunity to repair them. Children of alcoholics, like their parents, are isolated and typically bear shame, confusion, and guilt alone. Groups can provide children with a feeling that their experiences are not unique. Through participation in groups, children can learn to put the familial alcoholism into perspective, find ways to cope with it, and achieve satisfaction in life.

Introduction

For the past three years, the authors have been running an activities, play therapy group for the latency-age children of alcoholic parents. This article will discuss the effects of parental alcoholism on children's development during latency. These children represent a population at risk with a need for treatment by professionals who are knowledgeable about and comfortable with the discussion of alcoholism.

Kendra-Ann Brown, MSW, is Clinical Director of the Women's Alcoholism Program of the Cambridge and Somerville Program for Alcoholism Rehabilitation Inc., Cambridge, MA. Jeffrey Sunshine, M Ed., is former Counseling Intern with the Women's Alcoholism Program of the Cambridge and Somerville Program for Alcoholism Rehabilitation Inc., Cambridge, MA. Currently in private practice.

The Women's Alcoholism Program of the Cambridge and Somerville Program for Alcoholism Rehabilitation, Inc., Cambridge, MA, is a comprehensive treatment facility for alcoholic women and their families. Services include residential treatment, outpatient services, consultation and education.

Rationale

For the purposes of this paper, we will assume alcoholism to be a process characterized by repetitive abusive drinking, personality changes while drinking, and/or the individual's own declaration that s/he is an alcoholic. We further assert that this process exists independent of any underlying personality disorder. Finally, we contend that alcoholism affects not only the individual but the entire family unit.

As family therapists recognize, the family is an interactional system wherein each member affects the whole. The family of an alcoholic is constantly striving to achieve and maintain homeostasis, and thus adjusts around the alcoholism. The family members develop a crisis mentality and allow the drinking behavior to run their lives (Dulfano, 1978).

Life in an alcoholic family is neither consistent nor predictable (Fine, Yudin, Holmes, & Heineman, 1975). Everyday needs are ignored in the face of the alcoholic's numerous crises. The family accommodates these crises, which become a way of life. This gives the family a distorted view of the world. Affection, as well as sources of self-esteem and fun, are scarce commodities.

Because alcoholism carries with it a powerful social stigma, the alcoholic individual is often in denial about his or her problem. Frequently the family colludes with this denial. When the alcoholic family member is a woman, the denial is greatly exacerbated on the part of both the woman and her family (Sandmaier, 1980). Even when denial is not pronounced, the family frequently resists seeking treatment because of the shame and guilt involved in admitting to the alcoholic drinking. Therefore, alcoholism is often a closely guarded family secret which must be maintained at all costs. Sometimes the cost involves the distortion of reality and the use of incorrect labeling of behavior (Mommy is sleepy, ate something that made her sick, etc.). To a child, this process can greatly impede the development of reality testing. At other times, the secret is disclosed within the family but kept from the outside world. To do this, the family must become a closed system with rigid and impermeable boundaries. Family members become furtive and avoid close emotional contact with others. For the child to disclose the secret outside of the family can have disastrous consequences for her or him. It can involve risking parental disapproval or punishment, peer rejection, and/or possibly the destruction of family integrity by opening up the system to scrutiny. To the outside world, the family may look like any other on the block. Non-alcoholic members may become super-competent as a reaction formation against feelings of helplessness and low self-esteem. It is not unusual, for example, to find that the child voted "most likely to succeed" has an alcoholic parent (Black, 1981).

There are also often special problems for female alcoholics. "Studies show that men are significantly more likely to leave their alcoholic spouses than are women . . ."(Sandmaier, 1980). Therefore the child of an alcoholic mother must often deal with the double stigma of problem drinking and marital separation. Of those husbands who remain with their alcoholic wives, many are heavy drinkers themselves (Corrigan, 1980).

Latency-age children of alcoholic parents comprise a particularly vulnerable group, for several reasons. First, they must deal with the physical or emotional absence of the non-alcoholic parent and the effects of alcoholism on the total family system, including the lack of a consistent environment. Additionally, they learn to subjugate their needs so that they can fulfill roles in the family system that may have been vacated by the adults. Because the thinking of latency-age children is fairly concrete, their concepts of causal relationships are often distorted and tinged with magical thinking (Lidz, 1968). Sometimes they feel that they are directly responsible for family problems, such as divorce and alcoholism. Self-blame is often reinforced by the alcoholic's excessive use of externalization and projection to rationalize the drinking behavior: (If I didn't have these kids, I wouldn't need to drink so much.). One of the most tragic consequences of alcoholism is the fact that children of alcoholic parents have a much greater likelihood of developing alcoholism in later life than do children of non-alcoholic parents (Chafetz, Blane, & Hill, 1971).

Unfortunately, there are far too few places where a child can discuss parental alcoholism and obtain some relief from the shame and isolation resulting from keeping the family secret. Many alcoholism treatment programs and the self-help programs (Al-Anon; Alateen) do not usually provide services to preadolescent children, and the agencies that traditionally serve children, such as mental health and child guidance centers, often lack personnel trained in the differential diagnosis and treatment of alcoholism in the family (Weir, 1970).

Children are affected in different ways and to varying degrees by the presence of alcoholism in the home, depending on such factors as the child's age at onset of the alcoholism; the relationship with the alcoholic parent independent of the drinking behavior; the child's resources outside of the family; the availability of the non-alcoholic parent; and the child's innate endowment and basic constitutional makeup. It is, therefore, impossible to present a definitive profile of such a child; however, it is possible to make some generalizations from direct observation of these children. These generalizations will be made within the context of examining the ego tasks facing the latency-age child.

The Latency-Age Child and Familial Alcoholism

One of the primary tasks of latency is learning, which leads to mastery over the environment and increased self-esteem. Learning and related school activities (for example, sports and social clubs) facilitate the neutralization of aggression and the sublimation of the instinctual drives (Lidz, 1968). In order for optimum learning to take place a child needs a consistent environment that is adequate in affective nurturance and parental approval; a home atmosphere that is both intellectually stimulating and emotionally supportive and one in which basic biological needs are met. The atmosphere in alcoholic homes is frequently characterized by chaotic conditions, resulting in the child's being unable to concentrate on studies and, possibly in inconsistent eating and sleeping patterns. Furthermore, support and gratification of esteem needs are often inadequate. These factors help to explain the high incidence of learning problems among children from alcoholic homes (Chafetz, et al. 1971).

In order to mature and to prepare for the tasks of adolescence and young adulthood, the latency-age child must continue the process of separation and individuation begun in infancy. The child is expanding the world of object relations, and intense involvement with family is beginning to be moderated: closeness to peers is becoming increasingly important. In order to successfully negotiate this task, the child must feel that he or she moves away with the family's blessing, and that venturing into the world of external objects does not create a vacuum that can potentially destroy the integrity of the family.

As mentioned above, the family in which alcoholism is dynamic closes its walls and develops rigid boundaries in order to maintain its integrity and protect the family secret. The more rigid the family boundaries, the more difficult it is for members to move in and out freely. Children can play a variety of roles important to the homeostasis of the family. The family's need for the child to remain in these roles interferes with the ability to separate. Examples of these roles include a child being used as a scapegoat for the problems between the adults or as a substitute parent to help raise younger siblings and to assume household tasks.

Children need age-appropriate performance expectations and tasks that are realistically achievable in order to mature and develop healthy self-esteem. This self-esteem is, in turn, necessary for learning and for performing the other ego tasks required of the latency age child. Too much responsibility given to an unprepared child can result in such ego deficits as lack of tolerance for frustration, chronic feelings of helplessness and worthlessness, and a pseudomaturity that inadequately prepares the child for the tasks of adolescence and adulthood (Weir, 1970). This pseudomaturity robs a child of spontaneity and joy and isolates her or him from peers.

Latency is a time of considerable growth in the area of social development. Peers and teachers help the child to move away from the intense closeness to family of the early years and prepare him or her to take a place in the world as a social being. Shared secrets within the peer group and special clubs are an important part of the latency-age child's transition from child-in-family to more autonomous adolescent and later independent adult (Lidz, 1968). The child with an alocholic parent is inextricably bound to the family by the shared feelings of shame and efforts to camouflage the drinking behavior. It becomes difficult to withdraw an appropriate amount of cathexis from the family and to transfer it to peers. Furthermore, at a most basic level, children from alcoholic families are often unable to bring friends home because of the closed nature of the family system and because of the child's own embarrassment. These children may feel "different" from peers because of the nature of their home life; feeling different, they often become guarded and secretive, which greatly interferes with intimacy in peer relationships (Weir, 1970).

Children from alcoholic families are often prey to the full spectrum of emotional, behavioral, and learning disorders (Chafetz, 1971). Depression (often becoming manifest in adulthood) is a common neurotic manifestation (Black, 1981) and can result from the depriving nature of the environment, from the child's low self-esteem, and/or from the introjection of harsh and devalued parental objects. Fears and anxieties are also common and result from the lack of stability in the home and the resulting lack of inner security in the child. Problems often spill over into the classroom, where the whole spectrum of learning disorders may be observed. These include school phobia, inability to concentrate, learned helplessness, school failure and excessive activity. Behavioral and neurotic problems include acting-out and anti-social behaviors, e.g., stealing, lying, and excessive aggression; timidity and shyness and difficulty in sustaining relationships; excessive dependence, inability to share, and inordinate amounts of unneutralized rage in the face of frustration (Weir, 1970).

On the other side of this are children with precocious ego development, who have received recent attention in the literature under such labels as "Responsible One" and "Adjuster" (Black, 1981). These terms apply to children who defend against feelings of shame and inadequacy by making extraordinary achievements in the external world.

Therefore, children from alcoholic homes can be considered to be a population at psychological risk. They need therapy that is provided by people who are sensitive to the issues around the family's alcoholism and to the children's special needs. The authors contend that group settings provide this therapy well.

One of the primary tasks in the treatment of the latency-age child from an alcoholic home is to help the child bear the burden of the shameful and frightening family secret by bringing it out in the open. This process is immediately relieving to the child and causes her or him to feel less isolated. For this reason and because children from alcoholic homes often have deficits in the areas of social development and peer interaction, group is the treatment of choice.

Group Description

Our group is an activities-play therapy group for latency-age children (6-12 years), which has as its goal the dissemination of information about alcoholism and the repairing of relationships that may have been damaged in alcoholic families. Educating children about the disease removes the mystery surrounding it and provides a vehicle for the working through of feelings about parental alcoholism. The group meets during the school year for an hour each week, and children remain members for an average of two years. Group size is limited to eight members. Enrollment is open to children with either one or two alcoholic parents; the alcoholic parent is required to be in treatment (professional and/or self-help) for the alcoholism. Prior to acceptance, children are screened for any psychiatric/behavioral disorders that might make them inappropriate for group treatment. The group is heterogeneous with regard to age, sex, diagnosis, and socioeconomic class. The focus on alcoholism creates a group bond that transcends other differences; therefore this heterogeneity is effective.

The inclusion of siblings subgroups in the larger group has provided a unique opportunity for these children to work through family issues while simultaneously dealing with both group and individual issues. In alcoholic homes there is often little communication or support among family members. As channels of communication get opened up in the group, children find sources of support not only among other members but also in their own families.

The first few minutes of each group involve a social activity designed to help make the transition into the group. This might include encouraging the children to share something about themselves of which they are particularly proud and/or that has been difficult or painful for them.

The major portion of the hour consists of structured activity. Underlying the selection of these activities are the goals of providing alcohol education and fostering improved interpersonal skills. Providing education serves to demystify a taboo subject about which children have many fantasies. These fantasies often take the form of children blaming themselves for family problems. By presenting the concept of alcoholism as a disease with complex etiology, guilt is attenuated. Furthermore, factual information provides children with a sense of objectivity and intellectual mastery which allows them to cope with the chaotic conditions wrought by the alcoholism.

Another aspect of providing education is to help children deal with the inevitable feelings that are aroused by discussion of parental alcoholism. Examples of activities include puppetry, story telling, role playing, and films. Through these projective and educative activities, children can recognize, work through, and develop a more objective understanding of their parents' alcoholism. One activity often used is to show a film about an alcoholic family and have the children role-play it the following week, giving their own interpretations of the characters' feelings.

One common thread among children from alcoholic homes is that they perceive all drinking as bad, out of control, and constituting alcoholism. Therefore, included in our education is an explanation of the entire repertoire of drinking behaviors, including responsible drinking. Thus the child is dealing with factual and affective data about alcoholism.

Because alcoholism is a problem that affects the entire family, it is important to provide a forum in which the child can begin to communicate openly about it with the family. We provide such a forum by including the parents in the child's treatment. This involves a group for the parents, family conferences held at regular intervals, and an occasional group to which children may invite their parent(s).

Another important task of the group is to facilitate the child's development of healthy social interaction with both peers and leaders. The unpredictable environment and lack of consistent limits that characterize many alcoholic homes deplete the child's ability to trust other children and adults. We therefore try to establish a safe and trustworthy place by making the group predictable (dealing with vacations, holidays, terminations, etc.) and by developing rules, including the promise of confidentiality and a limit on aggression against others. We encourage children to replace aggression with appropriate assertion.

We have found that a group setting is a most effective means of treatment for children from alcoholic homes. Dealing with alcoholism as a group issue provides a universality of experience and reduces the feelings of the child's being the only one to whom this is happening. Groups have long been noted for their efficacy in dealing with interpersonal skills (Yalom, 1970) such as sharing, problem solving and communicating. Because of the frequent social isolation of children from alcoholic homes, group treatment fills a developmental need that might otherwise not be met.

REFERENCES

Black, C. Innocent bystanders at risk: The children of alcoholics. *Alcoholism: The National Magazine*, 1981, *1*(3), 22-26.

Chafetz, M. E., Blane, H. T., & Hill, M. J. Children of alcoholics: Observations in a child guidance clinic. *Quarterly Journal of Studies on Alcoholism*, 1971, *32*, 687-689.

Corrigan, E. M. *Alcoholic women in treatment*. New York: Oxford University Press, 1980.

Dulfano, C. Family therapy of alcoholism. In Zimberg, S., Wallace, J. & Blume, S. B. (Eds.), *Practical approaches to alcoholism psychotherapy*. New York: Plenum Press, 1978.

Fine, E., Yudin, L. W., Holmes, J. & Heineman, S. Behavior disorders in children with parental alcoholism. Paper presented at the Annual Meeting of the National Council on Alcoholism, Milwaukee, Wisconsin, April, 1975.

Lidz, T. *The person: His development throughout the life cycle*. New York: Basic Books, 1968.

Sandmaier, M. *The invisible alocholics: Women and alcohol abuse in America*. New York: McGraw-Hill, 1980.

Weir, W. R. Counseling youth whose parents are alcoholic: A means to an end as well as an end in itself. *Journal of Alcohol Education*, 1970, *16*(1), 13-19.

Yalom, I. D. *The theory and practice of group psychotherapy*. New York: Basic Books, 1970.

A GROUP TREATMENT APPROACH
FOR ADOLESCENT CHILDREN
OF ALCOHOLIC PARENTS

Joanne Deckman
Bill Downs

ABSTRACT. Alcoholism is a family disease, and children of alcoholics are considered at high risk for developing alcohol-related problems. It has been pointed out in recent literature that some of these children have emotional and behavioral problems; however, the majority may not develop such problems until adulthood. This paper describes a group counseling treatment modality for adolescents of alcoholic parents, with a goal of helping them with feelings of helplessness and isolation before they mature fully. The paper also describes various methods of providing a supportive atmosphere and improving communication skills. Results and common themes of the group experience are discussed.

Research data indicate that children of alcoholic parents are twice as likely to become alcoholic as children of non-alcoholic parents. Statistics indicate that 58 percent of this population become alcoholic, 30 percent marry alcoholics, and 12 percent have adjustment problems for years (Black, 1981). Furthermore, it has been estimated that there are a minimum of 28 million children of alcoholics (Black, 1981). Yet, "resources to meet the needs of the children are sadly lacking" (Hindman, 1976).

Alcoholism is a family disease. All members of an alcoholic home are psychologically, behaviorally, and socially affected. Most children of alcoholics are likely to experience an unstable family situation, often manifested by frequent parental quarreling and fighting. Frequently mentioned in the literature is the fact that children seem more emotionally upset by witnessing parental quarreling than by the excessive drinking itself (Wilson & Orford, 1978; Cork, 1969; Black, 1979). Black (1979) stated that over half of these children witness family violence, including physical threats and severe verbal abuse. The child's typical response is to withdraw,

---

Joanne Deckman, MA, CAC, is a social service worker for the Department of Children and Family Services, Chicago, IL. Bill Downs, MHS, is a counselor at the Alcoholism Out-Patient Treatment Center, Ingalls Hospital, Harvey, IL.

avoid, and ignore the alcoholic parent and sometimes the non-alcoholic one as well. Naturally the family atmosphere is very strained, and there is little communication and very few, if any, activities involving the whole family (Wilson & Orford, 1978).

As a result of this unstable family situation, certain psychological and emotional problems are likely to arise. Early exploratory research indicates that the children of alcoholics experience severe emotional and behavioral problems and underlying personality disturbances (Cork, 1969 ; Chafetz, Blane, & Hill, 1971). However, more recent evidence indicates that children of alcoholics are not necessarily more emotionally and behaviorally disturbed than children of non-alcoholics. Children of alcoholics do not easily fit into some particular or easily recognizable personality type, nor are they more likely to be emotionally disturbed (Kern et al, 1978). Black (1979) supports this view, stating that "the child with behavioral problems in the alcoholic home is in the minority." The early studies focused largely on "the problem child" and ignored possible differences between children of alcoholic fathers and alcoholic mothers. However, the report on a 20-year longitudinal study (Miller & Jang, 1977) indicated that the negative impact on children of an alcoholic mother is significantly greater than that of an alcoholic father.

It is generally agreed that children of alcoholic parents experience little genuine communication and expression of feelings. This is, of course, especially true of the child's interaction with the alcoholic parent, but can also be true for the non-alcoholic spouse, since a great deal of his or her time is spent trying to cope with the alcoholic. Black (1979) pointed out that even the responsible, bright, "well-adjusted" child has learned that it is not all right to express feelings like anger, sadness, or fear. Often, when these children want to talk at all they feel ignored. Pretty soon, they learn "not to feel." The negative consequences of this kind of family situation often do not become apparent until adulthood (Black, 1979).

The Therapy Group

Previous authors have mentioned the difficulty in recruiting adolescents for group therapy. The group addressed in this paper had the support of the Youth Services Program of the South Suburban Council on Alcoholism, in whose facilities the group was conducted. Most of the referrals come from within this department. Other referrals come from the Adult Outpatient Department, from responses to articles about the group appearing in the local paper, and from other local youth services agencies.

After an initial screening interview, each member was asked to make a commitment to the open-ended group for at least eight weeks. The core of the group consisted of three males and five females, ranging from 13 to 17 years of age. Four members lived with the alcoholic parent. Four of the alcoholic parents were actively drinking, and four were recovering. Only one of the alcoholic parents was the mother.

Both group leaders had completed formal education in alcoholism and counseling, and both worked together previously with younger children of alcoholics.

Goals

The goals of the group were (1) to provide education and information on the disease concept of alcoholism, addiction, effects of alcoholism on the family, enabling behavior, and alternative support groups such as Al-Anon, Alateen, and A.A.; (2) to provide a safe and supportive atmosphere; (3) to facilitate the identification and expression of feelings to help overcome feelings of isolation; (4) to improve communication skills within the family; and (5) to facilitate overcoming feelings of powerlessness and helplessness.

Methods

The educational material was interwoven within the group when relevant. This method was used to prevent a classroom-like atmosphere. A current film about alcoholism was shown and was followed with a discussion. Guest speakers from A.A., N.A. (Narcotics Anonymous), and Alateen also spoke to the group. The speakers were invited only after the approval of the group had been obtained.

Goals 2 and 3 above were achieved by providing a safe, supportive atmosphere. A client-centered, nondirective approach was taken, which seemed to work well. Identification of feelings was achieved through Rogerian and Gestalt techniques. As the group progressed, role playing and assertiveness training were employed to help the group members practice their new skills before using them in the family situation.

These children admittedly felt helpless to change anything in their families. Since feelings of helplessness are so prevalent in alcoholic families, we wanted them to experience their impact on the therapy group. It was made clear from the start that the group was theirs, and that the decisions made for the group were their responsibility. Rules for the group were kept to a minimum; the members initially spent part of one session working them out. However, the issue of rules periodically emerged in subsequent sessions.

Results and Discussion

After three months, an evaluation was distributed to seven members who were considered core members. The majority of the respondants rated the group "very good" or "excellent." According to them, the most helpful aspect of the group experience was overcoming feelings of isolation. Also noted as being very helpful was learning to share their problems and expressing their feelings with the other group members and with their families.

The facilitators' clinical impressions concur with the members' regarding overcoming feelings of isolation. It seems obvious that members gained a sense of universality from the experience. It appeared that the dominant emotional theme for this population was identifying and/or admitting anger and learning to appropriately express it. The immature denial of anger very much parallels the denial of anger in alcoholics. We feel that adolescent children of alcoholics display much more acting-out behavior than is indicated in the literature.

In general the participants seemed fearful to openly express the anger they were feeling and they often turned to various avoidance and/or distraction mechanisms while in group. Most often they were angry at the alcoholic parent, but sometimes also at the non-alcoholic parent. Role playing and assertiveness techniques are helpful in teaching adolescents how to appropriately express anger.

One session focused on the issue on confidentiality and trust. Because the female facilitator knew several of the childrens' parents, some members felt ambivalent about trusting her. This issue was brought to the foreground when the subject of smoking cigarettes in the group arose: members wanted to be able to smoke but were afraid this would get back to their parents. When the issue was dealt with, the trust issue was resolved.

The facilitators took a nondirective approach to a power struggle that developed between some group participants and the facilitators when rules were being discussed for the second time. Generally, the group displayed resistance toward rules, which seem to be experienced by children of alcoholics as a way of controlling their behavior. This issue relates strongly to their feelings of powerlessness and helplessness.

At the start of one session a female member adamantly wanted to reject a suggestion not to interrupt a member who was relating a personal problem. A number of members supported her; this sounded, again, too much like home or school. As the evening progressed, more and more distractions, avoidances, side conversations, and "goofing off" took place. To diffuse the power struggle, the leaders involved themselves together in a side discussion and did not attend to the group interaction. Later, a few participants expressed feelings of boredom. When the leaders rejected responsibility for the boredom, the participants assumed responsibility for group process. Participants eventually took on the responsibility for confronting any distracting behavior. The responsibility for what happened in the group was upon each member. Furthermore, as the members began to trust the fact that the leaders were willing to listen, offer support, and provide direction without controlling, they began to believe that it was truly their group.

Conclusion

It is the authors' belief that group counseling for adolescents of alcoholic parents is a valuable and effective means for overcoming feelings of isolation, for improving communication of feelings toward one another, for providing an atmosphere of support and caring, and for providing education concerning the disease of alcoholism. If viable prevention is to occur among this population, we feel that three areas must be addressed: (1) education about alcoholism as a disease; (2) the identification and appropriate expression of anger; and (3) overcoming feelings of powerlessness and helplessness.

REFERENCES

Black, C. Innocent bystanders at risk: The children of alcoholics. *Alcoholism,* Jan-Feb 1981, pp. 22–26

Black, C. Children of alcoholics. *Alcohol, Health and Research World,* Fall 1979, pp. 23–27.

Chafetz, M. E., Blane, H. T., & Hill, M. J. Children of alcoholics: Observations in a child guidance clinic. *Quarterly Journal on Studies of Alcohol,* 1971, *32,* 687–698.

Cork, M. *The forgotten children: A study of children with alcoholic parents.* Toronto: Alcoholism and Drug Addiction Research Foundation of Ontario, 1969.

Hindman, M. Children of alcoholic parents. *Alcohol, Health and Research World,* Winter 1975, p. 2.

Kern, J., Tippman, J., Fortgang, J., & Paul, S. R. A treatment approach for children of alcoholics. *Journal of Drug Education* 1977–1978, *7* (3), 207–218.

Miller, D., & Jang, M. Children of alcoholics: A 20-year longitudinal study. *Social Work Research and Abstracts,* 1977, *13*(4).

Wilson, C., & Orford, J. Children of alcoholics: Report of a preliminary study and comments on the literature. *Journal of Studies on Alcohol,* 1978, *39*(1), 121–142.

ALCOHOLISM TREATMENT FOR THE DEAF: SPECIALIZED SERVICES FOR SPECIAL PEOPLE

Paul Rothfeld

ABSTRACT. During the past decade, alcoholism treatment services in the United States have experienced unprecedented growth. The federal and local governments and the general public have become increasingly aware of the devastating impact of alcohol abuse and alcoholism on people's health and welfare and on the overall economy. As a result of this growing awareness, diversified alcoholism services are now available in communities throughout the country. Despite this preponderance of treatment, there is at least one segment of the alcoholic population which has been virtually unserved. This is the deaf alcoholic.

This paper will describe an innovative program of alcoholism treatment for the deaf.

First Contact with Deafness and Alcoholism

My first experience with deafness and alcoholism occurred in the summer of 1975, when a frustrated, distraught mother contacted me for assistance. Her thirty-year-old, prelingual, deaf son had developed a serious drinking problem accompanied by severe bouts of depression. He had just completed a three-week voluntary commitment at a state mental hospital, and his mother felt that his "treatment during that time consisted only of heavy sedation and locked wards." Apparently, as is so often the case, the hospital staff had little knowledge or understanding of deafness, and no specialized resources for the deaf were utilized.

At the mother's request, I met with the young man, Stephen Miller, to see if I could provide some help. My perceptions of deafness at that time were probably representative of a majority of the hearing population. I did not consider deafness one of the most debilitating handicaps; I felt sure that I could somehow communicate with the client; and as a recovered alcoholic

Paul Rothfeld is Executive Director, Cape Cod Alcoholism Intervention and Rehabilitation Unit, Inc., Pocasset, MA.

79

myself I felt sure there would be an immediate bond between us which would transcend all other barriers and allow a meaningful and effective therapeutic process to occur.

Barriers to Therapy

To some degree, all of the above conditions were true, and some positive interaction did occur at that first meeting and subsequent ones between myself and Steve. There definitely was some empathetic understanding on both our parts, and to some degree a trust relationship did develop. But always and ever, the barrier of our inability to communicate freely and easily blocked the path to a meaningful therapeutic process. The barrier became even more obvious to me when Steve and I attended an A.A. discussion meeting. A sign language interpreter was utilized and translated for Steve, as each person in the group participated in the discussion. It was impossible for Steve to keep up with the dialogue, let alone benefit from the often moving and personal testimony presented. I then began to understand and believe that if therapy was to be effective for the deaf, it should occur between peers. Deaf alcoholics should be in group process with other deaf alcoholics, and therapeutic dialogue should be direct from one group participant to another. I began to realize that a specialized program, uniquely designed to meet the needs of deaf alcoholics, was needed if people like Steve were to have a fighting chance to recover.

A Tragic Ending

During the next two years, I met with Steve on an on-and-off basis, more as a friend than as a therapist. He continually sought help through A.A., mental health services, and private practitioners, but all to no avail. Sadly and tragically, he ended his life on November 21, 1977. It is ironic that just twenty-one days earlier, I had completed and submitted an application to the NIAAA to fund a comprehensive program for deaf alcoholics. Although too late to help Steve, perhaps this new program would prevent a reoccurrence of so wasteful a loss of human life.

CCAIRU Project for the Deaf Becomes a Reality

On November 1, 1979, two years after my initial submission date to the NIAAA, the Cape Cod Alcoholism Intervention and Rehabilitation Unit (CCAIRU) Project for the Deaf became a reality, and the task at hand was to implement as quickly as possible the first comprehensive program for deaf alcoholics in the United States.

Project Staffing

The initial months of the first year were spent in trying to recruit staff with special skills in alcoholism and deafness. It became quickly evident that persons with knowledge and expertise in both areas were virtually non-existent. In fact, skilled therapists for non-alcoholic deaf persons are very few and are at a high premium in the job market. Once again, the underserved nature of the "hidden" deaf population is highlighted by the scarcity of skilled therapists available for a project of this type. The complex problems associated with deafness mandate that therapists have special knowledge and sensitivity in areas of deaf development and functioning, communication skills, linguistic retardation, and in intellectual, vocational, and psychiatric aspects of deafness.

As of early summer, 1980, fourteen staff positions have been filled by persons with diversified backgrounds supporting CCAIRU's multidisciplinary approach to alcoholism treatment. Six of these people are deaf themselves, and two are recovering alcoholics. One of the recovering alcoholic counselors is the child of deaf parents, and the other recovering alcoholic is herself deaf.

A staff requirement not experienced in the hearing world is the need for interpreters. In the original grant application, only one interpreter was included in the staffing pattern. It was naively believed that with all persons on staff being proficient in sign language, one interpreter would be sufficient. It became glaringly obvious that if a project for the deaf is to relate to the hearing world, interpreters are needed not only for clients, but also for deaf staff members. This very real problem besets most treatment programs for the deaf, both economically and in the availability of qualified personnel. By the summer of 1980, the CCAIRU Project for the Deaf had three permanent and three temporary interpreters working at its residential facility in West Falmouth, Massachusetts.

With a full complement of qualified staff, the CCAIRU Project for the Deaf was ready to accept clients to its residential facility on May 1, 1980. The facility has been named the Stephen Miller House in recognition of the young deaf alcoholic whose tragic quest for recovery was so instrumental in the development of the Project. An open house and dedication program was planned for October 4, 1980, and all persons interested in treatment for deaf alcoholics were invited to attend.

Widely Distributed Client Population

The incidence of alcoholism among the deaf is geographically widely distributed, and it is essential that an effective outreach and referral network be established on state and national levels so that accessibility for those in need of treatment can be assured.

During the first three months that the residential facility has been operational, approximately 50 percent of admissions have come from out of state, including Ohio, Michigan, Tennessee, and New Hampshire. To ensure that an efficient referral network is established on a nationwide basis, a National Advisory Board with broad geographical representation is being developed. It is hoped that this board will be instrumental not only in developing working referral affiliations nationwide, but also in documenting new knowledge gained in working with deaf alcoholics, so that it may be shared with others who plan similar ventures.

On a statewide basis in Massachusetts, a broad outreach and referral system is being developed with involvement by state agencies and consumer organizations that serve the deaf. Affiliation agreements have been entered into throughout the state with offices of the Department of Mental Health, the Massachusetts Rehabilitation Commission, and almost every alcoholism program in existence. As clients present themselves throughout Massachusetts, the CCAIRU Project for the Deaf, in close collaboration with affiliated agencies, will provide evaluation and placement in the residential program or in an outpatient service. It is planned that ultimately an outpatient/aftercare system will be operational, so that residents leaving the Stephen Miller House may continue in outpatient treatment upon return to their local communities. Comprehensive follow-up and continuing support are deemed essential for the deaf alcoholic returning to self-sustaining status as a member of the community-at-large.

Telephone Communications

It appears appropriate at this time to point out the very obvious but often overlooked fact that deaf people cannot communicate in the usual fashion over the telephone. Hence they have great difficulty in complying with that wonderful A.A. suggestion to "call before you pick up the first drink." There is a device which enables deaf people to communicate by telephone. It is known as a TTY (Telephone Typewriter), or more currently as a TDD (Telecommunication Device for the Deaf). As part of the CCAIRU treatment program, participants will be trained in the use of these devices (typing skills) and upon return to their homes will be assisted and encouraged to obtain a device through whatever sources are available. On a local level, the CCAIRU Project for the Deaf has installed a TDD at the County Emergency Medical Center, and the number is being publicized so that all deaf people on Cape Cod may benefit from this service. For the first time on Cape Cod, a deaf person in need of police, fire department, or emergency medical assistance can communicate directly with the emergency service center—if he or she has a TTD.

Treatment Program Content

The program consists of residential and outpatient components. Program content is similar to other traditional alcoholism programs and includes group and individual therapy, participation in A.A. meetings, vocational and educational planning, alcohol information, and general participation in the peer milieu.

There are significant differences, however, between a program for the hearing and a program for the deaf. These must be given careful recognition and attention if the program is to have positive results. The most significant area that needs to be continually addressed and worked on is that of communication skills. For a deaf person, language and vocabulary are frequently, if not invariably, comprehended and used on a much different level than for a hearing person with comparable intelligence. Staff must be continually aware that the meaning of many words may not be evident to deaf people. In written subject matter such as the A.A. books and pamphlets, much of the language is frequently not understood by deaf clients. Efforts have already been made to translate the 12 steps of A.A. into language that is more meaningful and more readily understood by the deaf.

A similar and equally complex problem is the varying levels of sign language proficiency by clients. In an early group of clients, one individual had no sign language skills whatsoever and could only read lips. As a consequence his early participation in group process was minimal. This was further complicated by his resistance in learning sign language, although this appeared to change gradually as he became more comfortable at the Stephen Miller House. Another client had extremely low-level signing skills, could not read lips at all, and had no verbal skills. He, too, was unable to participate effectively in group process, and counselors and/or interpreters had to be exceptionally proficient in order to communicate at a meaningful level with him. A related problem for staff with a client of this type is the difficulty in accurately assessing intelligence, aptitude, and possible psychiatric problems.

It is obvious that varying levels of language proficiency are a complex problem in the treatment of deaf clients. Effective ways of dealing with this problem must be developed if the treatment is to be viable and successful.

The CCAIRU Project for the Deaf is now fully operational and accepting clients for its residential program from all over the United States. The Stephen Miller House is a lovely, nineteen-room Victorian manse on four acres of land overlooking the waters surrounding Cape Cod. It provides a place where deaf alcoholics can participate in a program with peers and come to grips with their alcoholism and with the problems associated with deafness.

There is much to be learned about helping deaf alcoholics to recover from alcoholism. I am hopeful that the CCAIRU Project for the Deaf will make a significant contribution in pioneering the accumulation of this needed information while simultaneously providing help for those who enter its treatment program.

Author's Postscript—March, 1981

The Stephen Miller House, residential component of the Project for the Deaf, has now been fully operational for nine months. During this time, a variety of program and treatment approaches have been explored to determine the most effective methods for providing alcoholism treatment for deaf substance abusers with highly varied communication skills.

Involvement in A.A. is considered by most alcoholism programs to be an essential part of the recovery process. For some deaf clients, this is possible on a limited scale through the use of interpreters. In *all* cases, however, there is a definite reduction in full comprehension due to the differences in language perception between hearing and deaf people. In an effort to deal with this problem directly, clients and staff meet daily and endeavor to rewrite some of the A.A. literature so that it is more meaningful for the deaf. A.A. Steps One, Two, and Three are shown in Table 1 with the "translated" version for our clients alongside. It must be noted that this process is ongoing, and it is conceivable that eventually there will be three or four versions of each step, so that each person can select the most appropriate one.

Table 1: A.A. Steps and Translations for the Deaf

Original A.A. Step	Stephen Miller House Translation
Step 1: We admitted we were powerless over alcohol, that our lives had become unmanageable.	We say that alcohol beat me and we can't control what happens.
Step 2: Came to believe that power greater than ourselves had restored us to sanity.	We begin to have true feeling that not depend me alone to change me to sober life; not crazy, not drunk.
Step 3: Made a decision to turn our will and our lives over to the care of God as we understood him.	We decided to allow God or others to help how we live.

Additional creative programming is being developed in the area of art and drama therapy. In small groups, clients are asked to draw pictures that reflect their experiences as drinking alcoholics, as sober alcoholics, and as deaf human beings struggling in a hearing world. Each client then explains his or her drawing in mime or sign language. The pictures are then utilized for role play exercises, with participants taking turns acting out their own and other client's drawings. Response to this *visual* therapy has been most positive, with a high degree of feeling displayed, which was not previously evident in more traditional group process.

The task at hand is a most difficult and challenging one for both staff and clients. It demands creativity, flexibility, and willingness to frequently be wrong and start over. The rewards, however, are equally great, and the Project will persevere in its search for developing the most effective treatment possible for hearing impaired alcoholics and other substance abusers.

GROUP TREATMENT
FOR ELDERLY ALCOHOLICS
AND THEIR FAMILIES

Jean Dunlop
Barbara Skorney
James Hamilton

ABSTRACT. The use of treatment groups in a program for elderly alcoholics is described in this paper. The program is a demonstration project funded by a federal grant through the National Institute of Alcohol Abuse and Alcoholism. The project has as its objective the investigation of the extent of alcohol problems among the elderly and the development of effective treatment modalities for those who experience these problems. The treatment groups described are considered part of the continuum of treatment for alcohol problems that includes an aftercare group, a couples' counseling group, and a family group. Some characteristics unique to older persons and their families are found to be significant relative to the group process and content. These are described, as well as the changes that occurred in the groups as they evolved.

The Senior Alcohol Services Project for Elderly Alcoholics is a demonstration project funded by the National Institute for Alcohol Abuse and Alcoholism. The project has three major purposes: to determine the extent of the problem drinking in the over-60 population of Clark County, Washington; to provide training and information to the community about the problem of alcoholic drinking among the elderly; and to develop and implement effective treatment modalities to serve this population. The project treatment team includes a clinical psychologist, an alcoholism counselor, an outreach worker, and a medical social worker. The staff's major involvement with the clients has been in the motivational and aftercare phases of treatment.

Jean Dunlop, RN, MA, is a medical social worker, Barbara Skorney, MSW, is Project Director at Senior Alcohol Services, and James Hamilton, CAC, is a Certified Alcohol Counselor at Senior Alcohol Services, HWPC, Vancouver, WA.

Intervention

Group work for clients and their families has been highly effective at several points in the treatment continuum—in the motivational phase, in the intensive treatment period, and during aftercare. It is used as a powerful tool in a process called intervention during the motivational phase of treatment. Intervention was developed by the Johnson Institute to assist a potential client in recognizing and accepting the existence of a drinking problem. It is a structured event that brings together a group of family and other concerned persons in a carefully planned meeting with the client. Denial of the problem is a common defense mechanism employed by the problem drinker, and it often prevents him or her from accepting help offered. Frequently, confrontation by one person is ineffective, since the client easily rationalizes and manipulates to avoid accepting the facts presented. A structured intervention circumvents this problem. A counselor moderates the meeting, during which each person presents facts about the client's drinking-related behavior. Statements are made in a caring, concerned way. Angry accusations and blaming are avoided because they are counterproductive and lead to defensiveness and resistance. The value of group confrontation lies in the increased power of several caring persons expressing their concern about the client. This kind of pressure is frequently effective in motivating the person to seek help.

Planning for Aftercare

The client who has been motivated to accept is treatment usually admitted to a residential center for 21 to 30 days of intensive treatment. Group counseling is an important part of an intensive treatment program. In order to be effective with the older person, counselors need to be aware of the ways in which the elderly's responses differ from younger persons. Heavy confrontation is not effective with older persons. They have suffered a variety of losses whicn, when combined with the stigma of alcoholism, have damaged their self-image. Approaches that focus on the client's positive assets and strengths can help them regain control over their lives and instill hope for the future.

Aftercare planning begins prior to completion of the acute phase of treatment. During this transition, the project staff need to maintain a close relationship with the client, so that there is continuity of treatment. In cooperation with the treatment center counselor, the project staff and client develop an aftercare plan which addresses the client's need for continuing support in sobriety as well as other needs such as psychosocial, economic, and health. The need for a comprehensive, holistic approach in the aftercare phase is important. Aftercare plans are individualized, and clients may participate in the aftercare program as long as needed.

Need Met by Aftercare Groups

The effectiveness of the aftercare group has been dramatically demonstrated. Persons attend this group for a variety of reasons: most take part initially because the group is perceived to be a place to receive direction and support for sobriety from project staff and fellow recovering problem drinkers. A few persons have been court-mandated to attend, but most have come of their own volition. Some have felt pressure to attend by treatment center and/or project staff. Whatever the reason, once group involvement occurs, the majority of members express surprise and delight at the atmosphere of friendliness and warmth they find. Most clients had become socially isolated and depressed during the progression of their drinking career, with a resultant lessening of self-confidence and self-esteem. These feelings may reflect today's youth-oriented culture, the life losses suffered by the older person, or the stigma placed upon alcoholism by the elderly. The acceptance new members receive from others in the group is highly rewarding and seems to prompt continuing attendance.

The group meets several other needs, also. With regular attendance and renewed self-confidence, social skills return. The aftercare group also provides an important opportunity for clients to reminisce about their life experiences. Reminiscence helps older persons to "make some sense out of" their lives and to give their existence value and meaning. The need for fun and relaxation is met as members receive encouragement and positive reinforcement for sobriety. Often there is considerable joking and hilarity along with serious discussion.

Although the social functions of the group have been important, the major therapeutic contribution of the group process has been to teach older clients how to disclose their feelings to others. Many older persons were taught not to express their feelings as they were growing up. Members often have bottled up feelings for years, and they find real catharsis when they express resentments, fears, and loneliness. This release is enhanced by the feeling of commonality in the group and the realization that one is not alone in the experience of such feelings.

Education in Aftercare

As the group has evolved, the project staff has felt that educational sessions would benefit members. When left to its own devices, the group basically functions as a social group. It meets the needs described above, i.e., the need for acceptance, the need to develop social skills and retrieve self-esteem, the need for reminiscing, the need for fun and relaxation, and the need to release feelings. Although the latter is gently but purposefully encouraged by project staff, the other results are the inadvertent outcome of the unguided group process.

The dilemma of how to structure the group to meet the staff's agenda and the members' perceived needs has been resolved successfully as follows: the group continues to meet for 1½-hour sessions at twice-weekly intervals. Once a week the first half hour is used for educational presentations. Topics have included a series on Transactional Analysis, a series on the twelve steps of A.A., a series on assertiveness training, sessions on the use of medication, nutrition, physical fitness, grief resolution, relaxation techniques, depression, sexuality, family dynamics, and feelings. Members then divide into small counseling groups, which last about 45 minutes. The final 15 minutes are set aside as a social time when the groups join together for coffee, cookies, and conversation. On the other meeting day each week, the counseling groups meet for one hour and the final half hour is spent socializing. Members seem content with this system, and the group membership has continued to grow. Since time and space are flexible, persons can linger for longer socializing if they are so inclined.

The Elderly and The Group Process

Some characteristics unique to the elderly have affected the group process, and to some degree, the content of the group sessions. Members may have physical impairments, which need to be recognized and accommodated. The meeting room has to be accessible to people using wheelchairs, canes, and walkers. Members prefer daytime meetings; they do not like to travel at night. Hearing difficulties are common, so it is necessary to speak slowly and distinctly to be understood. Most members wear glasses and find large print helpful. It is necessary for the therapist to be especially aware of the jargon used in the mental health and alcoholism fields. Such a word as "stroke" (a Transactional Analysis term meaning a unit of recognition) has meant a medical event to more than one older client. "I" messages may be interpreted as "eye" messages and "growth" either stops at 21 or is removed by a surgeon. The group as a whole is reluctant about and embarrassed at self-disclosure, although, with repeated contacts and the development of trust and rapport, this can be overcome. The elderly generally dislike profanity. Social amenities are observed as a matter of course. Members also enjoy being with a group of peers. Many speak of the difficulty they have relating to the younger persons in the mixed age groups they have encountered in treatment centers and in self-help groups. Most relate easily, however, to the spiritual emphasis they find in A.A. One of the most positive aspects of the aftercare group is the support and encouragement members give to each other.

Couples' Counseling

Another effective treatment modality for elderly alcoholics and their families has been the couples' counseling group. This group is composed of three to five older couples and meets once a week. Major foci of this group are the development of self-awareness and the improvement of communication patterns between mates. Some Transactional Analysis is used and, occasionally, gestalt techniques. Assertiveness training concepts are presented, and members practice new behavior using role play and role reversal. Appropriate expression of feelings is a common goal in these sessions. The members respond positively to the commonality they feel in hearing their own experiences echoed by others.

Family Meetings

A successful group experience in the project is the weekly family meeting. The purpose of this group is twofold: to educate the family about alcoholism, and to make members aware of the way in which they adjust to the problem drinking. The group is also used to ventilate feelings and has thus evolved into a support group for members. One very frequent characteristic is an overwhelming feeling of guilt. This seems compounded in the adult children of alcoholic clients, who feel responsible for their elderly parent and his or her drinking. An added complication is the fact that many clients do indeed have physical and mental impairments and have a legitimate need for help. Practical issues such as problem-ownership and feelings of responsibility are addressed in discussions. Typically, these individuals "parent" the drinking mother or father, leading to even greater feelings of inadequacy and worthlessness on the part of the parent. Through the meetings, they realize their inability to control another's behavior. Family relationships and communication patterns begin improving even in cases where the drinking does not stop.

Individual Family Counseling

Individual family counseling sessions were started as an outgrowth of the family meeting. Although most of the project's clients are retired, some are married to younger women and still have teenage children at home. These youths and their parents have problems typically found in younger alcoholic families. Problems addressed in these sessions include ineffective and damaging communication patterns. The therapist helps the family identify problems and makes an initial diagnosis. Problem-solving techniques—definition of the problem, who owns the problem, how to develop options to solve the problem, and how to try an option—are taught. The therapist emphasizes communication skills, and there are sessions on active listening and assertiveness. Role reversal has been an effective technique for illustrating poor communication patterns. Families that combine the multiple problems of alcoholism, retirement, and disability have responded well to family counseling sessions.

Summary

Group work is a basic component of treatment in the Senior Alcohol Services Project. It has proven effective and efficient in motivational counseling, intensive treatment, in aftercare, and with families. Elderly problem drinkers respond as positively to group counseling as do their younger counterparts if the unique characteristics of the elderly are addressed.

REFERENCES

Bengtsen, Vern L., *The Social Psychology of Aging*, Indianapolis: The Bobbs-Merrill Co., Inc., 1980.

Butler, Robert N. and Lewis, Myrna J., *Aging and Mental Health*, Saint Louis: C.V. Mosby Co., 1977.

Mishara, Brian L. and Kastenbaum, Robert, *Alcohol and Old Age*, New York: Grune and Stratten, 1980.

FILMS

Minneapolis: Johnson Institute; "The Enablers" and "Intervention".